Also by Wendy Schlessel Harpham, M.D.

DIAGNOSIS: CANCER
YOUR GUIDE THROUGH THE FIRST FEW MONTHS

AFTER CANCER

___

A GUIDE TO YOUR NEW LIFE

AFTER CANCER

A GUIDE TO YOUR NEW LIFE

Wendy Schlessel Harpham, M.D.

W·W·Norton & Company

New York   London

The text of this book is composed in 12/14 Berkeley Old Style Book,

with the display set in Gill Sans Condensed Roman.

Composition and manufacturing by the Maple-Vail Book

Manufacturing Group.

Book design by Margaret M. Wagner.

Library of Congress Cataloging-in-Publication Data

Harpham, Wendy Schlessel.

After cancer : a guide to your new life / Wendy Schlessel

Harpham.

p.   cm.

Includes bibliographical references and index.

1. Cancer—Popular works.   2. Cancer—Miscellanea.

3. Cancer—Psychological aspects.   I. Title.

RC263.H359   1994

616.99′4—dc20   93-44553

ISBN 0-393-03664-2

W. W. Norton & Company, Inc.

500 Fifth Avenue, New York, N.Y. 10110

W. W. Norton & Company Ltd.

10 Coptic Street, London WC1A 1PU

1 2 3 4 5 6 7 8 9 0

For Ted

Our knowledge about cancer is constantly changing. This book is not intended as a substitute for competent medical care. It serves to supplement the information provided by your doctors and nurses.

Contents

7

Prologue

My final chemotherapy treatment was a breeze. The nurse deftly slipped the needle into a hidden vein. The brew of chemicals slowly flowed into my body as it had for the previous fifteen treatments. As the last ounce disappeared from the bag, the needle was withdrawn from my hand and a Band-Aid was placed over the puncture site. My nurse gave me a big hug, exclaiming, "It's over. You're done with your chemo." Although dazed from the antinausea medications, I felt good. My husband, Ted, and I left the treatment room for the last time.

Seven months earlier, in November 1990, I had been hospitalized with severe leg and back pain. My life had been dramatically and unalterably changed when surgery revealed lymphoma. After years of practicing internal medicine in my solo practice, with my children a few months shy of two, four, and six years old, I had become a cancer patient.

During the months of my cancer treatments, I experienced the baldness, fatigue, and nausea, as well as the emotional roller coaster of fear and confidence, anxiety and calm, depression and elation, that many cancer patients know. Cancer taught me about myself, my faith, my family, my priorities, the richness of friendships, and the fragility of life. I worked hard to squeeze every possible good out of my time with cancer, and to learn as much as I could about being a patient, so that I could be a better doctor when I was done with cancer.

Unfortunately, being done with chemotherapy did not mean I was done being a patient. After my last chemotherapy treatment, my blood counts dropped toward zero, as they had after every treatment. In addition to the expected fatigue and poor appetite, I developed an inflamed vein in my arm. I was hospitalized to receive intravenous antibiotics. The vein did not improve and had to be removed. Finding myself in the operating room was like a bad dream; I was once again sick and a full-time patient wondering when I would regain control of my life. I lay on the cold, hard table, my bald head covered with my favorite fuchsia scarf. The beeps of my heart monitor provided the background rhythm as I watched the pathologist, my friend Pam, catch the culprit, worm-like clotted vein in her basin.

As it turned out, the vein was sterile, the intravenous antibiotics were stopped, and I was discharged from the hospital the same night. Events over the next few weeks enticed me to believe that I would finally have a quick slide back to a normal life. My blood counts drifted up out of the danger zone for the last time, and I began to socialize. My scalp grew a shadow of brown fuzz, enough for Ted to call me Rapunzel. More important, a series of tests and scans showed that there was no sign of cancer anywhere. We had achieved complete remission.

The euphoria and sense of rebirth lasted a few days, but soon I could not avoid the next big decision: what to do to maximize my chance of maintaining my remission. Ted and I talked with my doctors. We read articles and books about my type of lymphoma. We arranged for a second-opinion consultation with a lymphoma specialist at the Dana Farber Cancer Center in Boston.

I was very anxious before the consultation. I was afraid he would find some spot of cancer missed at my reevaluation. I also harbored the more rational fear that, in his opinion, my best chance for a durable remission would be to undergo extensive radiation or a bone marrow transplant. Almost as much as I wanted to do the right thing, I wanted my bout with cancer to be over and to get back to a normal life. But it was not over, not yet anyway.

After arriving in Boston, with our three children spoiled safely with their grandparents, Ted and I walked Freedom Trail like all the other tourists. Unlike the others, I waited at the entrance when everyone else looked at the historic grave sites. Gazing at tombstones, pondering mortality, made it impossible for me to repress concerns about the upcoming consultation.

Ted and I ate lunch at a famous seafood restaurant, where we were ushered to a long, community table. All the other diners appeared caught up in their enjoyment of food and family, while I had the surreal feeling that I was watching myself from a distance. Ted relished the clams, encouraging me to taste just one. I declined, my appetite still poor from the chemo. That evening, in our romantic little hotel room, we both silently wondered whether the next day would be the beginning of more upheaval or the conclusion of a difficult chapter of our life. I slept well that night, while Ted spent the night in the bathroom, sick to his stomach. We were both glad I had not taken him up on his clam offering.

The consultation at the cancer center went well. Despite my devil's advocate role, the doctor told us what we had hoped to hear: his recommendation for me was no further treatment. He reassured me that my fatigue was not unexpected after intensive chemotherapy and that it would improve. My persistent leg and back pain was probably due to nerve damage from the months when my cancerous lymph nodes had pressed on the nerves to these areas. All in all, I was in an excellent position to start my journey back to a normal life.

Despite my enviable circumstances—enviable, that is, for your average chemo patient—I was far from being normal. After we returned to Dallas, I was more anxious and less happy than I had been before I got sick. Even though I had been off all chemotherapy and antibiotics for weeks, I developed antibiotic-associated colitis, a condition that caused diarrhea, nausea, and a generally sick feeling. I started to speed-walk for exercise, but the more I did, the more my leg and back hurt. Having exercised my entire life, I figured that I just had to walk through the pain to get back in shape. Exercise was part of who I was. If I worked out, I was healthy. And I wanted desperately to be healthy again. So I worked out and hurt. My appetite was still poor, and eating continued to be a chore. I lost ten pounds in four weeks. Would I ever enjoy eating again? Would I ever feel like my old self again?

Time was ticking away. The doctors with whom I shared responsibility for patient care on the weekends (my "call partners") wanted to know when I was going to be back at work. I was used to planning for every contingency, so it was very distressing not to know when the diarrhea would quit for good, when the pain would lessen, or when my appetite and stamina would return. I tried to be optimistic, telling myself, "I will be better tomorrow," but I just wasn't.

Expecting to feel awful with chemo made the discomforts more bearable. Expecting to feel good when it was over made relatively minor discomforts intolerable. What made it worse was that everyone around me seemed to think I should be feeling great and doing well now that my chemo was over.

And despite my remission, my home life unraveled. Dealing with my kids was a strain for me. Although I was immensely grateful to be with them, I felt guilty and upset when I was too tired to deal with their normal squabbles and shenanigans. I was supposed to have learned something deep and meaningful about life from my cancer. Why was I bothered by their spilled glasses of milk?

No longer a chemo patient, I assumed more responsibilities at home. Unfortunately, I could not figure out how much responsibility I could manage, how much rest I needed. If Ted tried to give me extra help, I was upset that he did not think I was well enough to take care of things. If he left things for me to do, I was upset that he did not realize how exhausted I was.

Ted justifiably became very irritable, and our relationship became strained. His own emotional and physical reserves were depleted. Now that I was out of immediate danger, all of the fears and anxieties that Ted had kept submerged during my treatments were bubbling to the surface. And he was distressed about all the time he had lost from his own work as a professor of political economy. He worried about money, which made me worry about money. Ted, my chief support person, needed a break from supporting.

Yet I still needed him. I needed his support after a tense discussion with my call partners about returning to work, after I declined offers to help out with the children's school events, as I tried to establish a new routine in my day. I found all of the daily big and little decisions stressful. After I had dealt gracefully with hundreds of decisions prior to my cancer, seeing myself stressed by these decisions was itself stressful. Life was not what we expected after cancer.

Recognizing that things were bad, Ted and I did what we had always done: we talked and listened to each other. We analyzed our situation until we felt we couldn't sneeze without analyzing it. We realized that underlying all of our stress, all of our anxiety about our work, kids, time, and money, was the reality that we had dodged a bullet. The painful reality for Ted was that he could not protect us from the threat of my illness. The painful reality for me was that I was not yet well.

We both had to accept, however reluctantly, just how different I was after cancer, physically and emotionally. Our old patterns and expectations no longer applied. We both had to sort through all the changes and what they meant.

I am a problem solver who wants immediate answers, and I knew I needed outside help. "Dialogue," the hospital's cancer support group, became an important place for validating my feelings and for receiving caring, practical advice. In addition, individual counseling with the hospital's social worker saved me months of working through the issues by myself.

Ted and I were both cancer survivors, and we both had to learn how to cope with the fears and anxieties. Understanding this helped us help each other through this awful time.

After a six-week delay because of the colon problems and fatigue, three and a half months after my last treatment, I reopened my practice part-time. My appetite was returning. Chili tasted like chili, chicken tasted like chicken, ice cream tasted like ice cream, and they all tasted good. My hair was growing in curly and thick, nicer than my prechemo hair. My energy was returning. As I became a regular fixture at the hospital again, the commotion of reacquaintance with my colleagues became less and less frequent. I felt that life was getting back to normal.

Except for the persistent leg and back pain. Five months after my chemotherapy was completed, my internist recommended further evaluation of the pain. I declined, saying, "I'm not scared that I have cancer again. I'm just all doctored out. I can not face more doctors, more tests, more medicines right now." Enabling me to retain some control, my internist agreed for the time being to postpone any workup.

The one-year anniversary of my diagnosis was approaching. My lymph nodes remained small, but my leg pain was worse. It was the exact same pain that I had had when I was diagnosed with cancer, and it taunted my intense desire to put my patienthood behind me. Intellectually, I did not think it could be due to a recurrence of the cancer. Besides, since the day I was diagnosed, I had promised myself that I was not going to be like one of those patients who forever worried about a recurrence every time they had a little ache or cough. I had told this to Ted, my doctors, my friends, and anyone else who would listen. I believed it. I believed it until I found myself again in the CAT scanner, probably one of the only doctors to know that there is a little happy face handdrawn on the inside of the scanner's big ring, where only the patient can see it. The hum of the scanner was horribly familiar, like a recurring nightmare.

I resembled almost all other survivors of serious cancers—I, too, was afraid of recurrence. My doctor's white coat no longer set me apart. Again, I reluctantly accepted that I was still a patient. This new level of acceptance liberated me to find ways to cope.

I agreed to see the neurologist about my pain. On the anniversary of my cancer diagnosis, the neurologist confirmed nerve damage. He predicted that resolution of the pain, if it ever resolved, would take months to years. It was bittersweet affirmation that the bigger problems of cancer and chemotherapy were resolved.

Leg pain due to nerve damage was a health problem like any other that normal people can have. But I was different: I had had cancer. When other symptoms or problems popped up, rationally or irrationally, fleetingly or obsessively, depending upon the problem, I thought of recurrence. I thought of new problems I could develop from my cancer treatments.

Even when cancer was not an issue, going to the doctor was. Appointments, examinations, tests, and medicines all reminded me of a time that I would rather have forgotten. Just the thought of being evaluated pounded on the still-soft shield of safety I was rebuilding.

Subconsciously, we all build shields to feel safe. These illusionary shields allow us to function effectively. Major trauma such as rape, accidental maiming, or a personal brush with life-threatening illness breaks down your shield. With time and effort, you rebuild it, but you are forever different and your shield is never as solid. In one important way cancer is a trauma different from other traumas: cancer can come back. If I was ever going to feel normal again, I was going to have to find healthy ways to deal with my fear of recurrence.

Yet this fear was only one of the changes accompanying recovery from cancer treatment. My search for knowledge and understanding of these changes encouraged me to grow strong from this painful recovery process, much as white light passing through a prism emerges as a rainbow on the other side.

I found the months after cancer at least as challenging as the months with cancer. It was a transition period during which the physical and emotional aftereffects of cancer treatment slowly disappeared or reached a plateau that helped to define the new me.

In one crucial way, how I coped after cancer was more important than how I coped during cancer: my physical and emotional recovery would affect the quality of my life forever. How I recovered from my cancer experience would shape my new concept of "normal."

My attitude toward all of the changes, problems, and losses of my recovery was similar to my attitude toward living with cancer and chemotherapy: I could not choose my circumstances, but I could choose the way I faced them. I talked with people who by personal or professional experience had found ways to cope with cancer, and even prosper. I focused on what I gained from my experience of illness. The one thing I could not do was ignore the fact that I had been a cancer patient or that I was recovering from cancer treatment.

As I came to recognize the importance of the process of recovery, the physician-observer in me watched my family's struggles and my response. I went to my computer to record and make sense of my personal observations and the information available in the literature. Writing had always been an effective coping style for me. Struggling through recovery was no different.

While going through my chemotherapy, I wrote a book, *Diagnosis: Cancer: Your Guide through the First Few Months*. The writing was fun and healing; the editing was tedious and draining. As *Diagnosis: Cancer* neared readiness for publication, the business details overwhelmed any sense of creativity. Like a woman in labor vowing that she would never get pregnant again, I vowed that I would never write another book.

Yet once *Diagnosis: Cancer* was published, I was gratified by seeing how it helped others. And if my basically solid family was hitting rough times after cancer, then other families probably had it even rougher. I had to write this book. After all, I am a doctor. Helping others is what I do.

I started taking notes for *After Cancer*. A book on this subject was a great challenge because books and articles about recovery from cancer treatment are fewer and less accessible than those about the physical and emotional aspects of active cancer and cancer treatment. Transforming my notes into a book suitable for survivors of cancer was my way of giving back after being given so much. If this book helps even one other person get through the time after cancer more easily, writing it will have been worth it.

As it turned out, writing *After Cancer* helped me through many cancer- and treatment-related medical problems and emotional issues that occurred during the writing. An understanding of the facts and philosophies presented in *After Cancer* helped me cope with two recurrences of my lymphoma and the closing of my beloved medical practice. Preparing and writing *After Cancer* enabled me to reach a new equilibrium, a new peace. Coping with cancer has been and will continue to be an ongoing, ever-changing process for me. I loved my life before I got cancer, but I can never go back to where I was. Not physically or emotionally. Today swollen lymph nodes, rashes, and backaches engage my attention. Carpooling, exchanging hugs, and caring for my patients are cherished privileges. Traffic jams, spilled milk, and crayoned walls are of no consequence.

Awareness of life's limits has expanded my sense of time by encouraging me to appreciate each and every day. Cancer has taught me how to live fully in the present. In learning to cope with cancer, I acquired tools for living that ease hard times and add sparkle to the mundane. Many good things have happened to me since I was first diagnosed with cancer. Never would I choose to have cancer, but I truly love my life better after cancer than before.

After cancer the prospect of a normal life is an alluring goal. "I just want to lead a normal life again." For most survivors, however, it is impossible to go back to where they were before cancer. To have a normal life after cancer means creating a new normal that incorporates the physical, emotional, and spiritual changes catalyzed by your cancer experience. Use this book as a guide to your new life.

Introduction

You know what it is like to be told you have cancer. You have been through evaluation and treatment. The shock and all-encompassing drama surrounding your diagnosis and cancer therapy are fading or long gone. Whether your cancer treatments are near completion or have been finished for a while, you feel that it is time to get back to normal.

You are a cancer survivor, someone who has been diagnosed with cancer and is still alive. Cancer survivors include those who have just been diagnosed, those who were cured of cancer decades earlier, those who have been living with cancer for years, as well as those in terminal stages of an unresponsive cancer. Whether or not you like it, "survivor" is the accepted term used in lay and professional publications to identify people who have or had cancer. The value of this definition of cancer survivor is that it confers more hope and dignity than "cancer victim" or "cancer patient."

If you are one of the luckiest survivors, there is no evidence of your cancer and you need no further treatment. Others of you had cancer that responded to treatment, but you will need additional cancer treatment for a very long time, if not for the rest of your life. Still others of you have been through cancer treatments only to learn that you will probably be living with cancer from now on.

The cancer experience is different for each person. For some of you, cancer was a minor intrusion that did not produce all the emotional overtones that usually accompany a cancer diagnosis. For example, if you had a cancerous mole removed in a twenty-minute surgery, leaving a three-inch scar hidden by your clothes, followed by one day's worth of scans and blood tests that declared you "cured," your life probably continued as usual with barely a skipped beat. Few people were involved with your scare. Like all cancer patients, you still need to be seen and examined periodically for signs of recurrence, but your cancer history has little impact on your day-to-day life.

Others of you have been through intensive chemotherapy followed by a bone marrow transplant. You may have been in the intensive care unit for part of your treatment. Your surviving at all may have been in doubt. Everyone who knows you is aware that you have been battling cancer. It has been a long time since you lived life as you knew it before your illness. It is going to be yet another long period of time before you feel normal, physically or emotionally. Your cancer experience affected every fiber of your being.

Most cancer survivors fall somewhere in the middle. You have been through some combination of treatment, either surgery and/or radiation and/or chemotherapy and/or biological therapy. Many of you have sustained permanent physical losses—a breast, a lung, an arm, your face, your voice, your intellect. More of you are experiencing temporary physical losses—your energy, your hair. Most of you have found being a cancer patient emotionally unsettling at best, devastating at worst.

Whatever your path to where you are today, you are all at the threshold of a journey to your new life, to a new normal. By "normal" I mean that, as in your life before cancer, there is some predictable pattern to your days and weeks, you have a life outside of your cancer and cancer treatments, your activities and goals are matched to your abilities and desires, and you are focused on the life you are living. Some of you aim to resume where you left off, while others of you choose to make major changes in your personal or professional life. Still others of you have no choice about major changes you have to make. Most of you relish the thought of returning to normal, any normal.

Recovery after cancer treatment is different from adjustment to a new diagnosis and dealing with cancer treatment. When you were first diagnosed with cancer, you and your family were expected to need information and support. Hotlines, referral centers, libraries, bookstores, and various newsletters supplemented the one-on-one information and support provided by your medical team. Your knowing friends, family members, clergy, and co-workers expected you to have special needs. During your crisis of cancer you were expected to need the busy doctors' and nurses' precious time.

Now suddenly your cancer treatments are over, or you have been placed on maintenance therapy. It is difficult to find information about recovery from cancer treatment. Your friends, family members, clergy, and co-workers do not know what to expect from you, or they seem to expect you to be your old self. Your doctors and nurses are busy tending to patients in crisis, patients with needs that you understand because you were a patient in crisis yourself just a short while ago. How do your seemingly less serious needs fit in to the ever-busy schedules of the doctors and nurses?

This book will help you and your family get through the transition to your new life as easily and safely as possible. It will help you understand and deal with many of the physical, social, and emotional problems that tend to accompany recovery from cancer treatment. Like *Diagnosis: Cancer,* this book has two underlying philosophies: knowledge is power, and there are always choices. "Knowledge is power," a cliché for marketing everything from business courses to magazine subscriptions, is a gem of truth in the context of cancer. Knowledge is good for you. It allows you to participate in your care and be your own best advocate. Knowledge will provide you with the tools you need to cope with the changes and problems after cancer treatment. These tools will help you regain some control, avoid or minimize emotional and physical pain, and look to your future in a more positive and productive way.

You cannot choose that you had cancer and that you may have cancer- and treatment-related problems. You *can* choose how you deal with your cancer history. You can choose how any changes and problems affect you medically, emotionally, and socially.

A key ingredient for coping and growing through adversity and recovery is the belief that there is always hope. Nourishing hope will enable you to use your knowledge to prevent or minimize problems related to your cancer.

This book provides a very basic and general framework for understanding and exploring what is happening to you as you recover from cancer treatment. It suggests ways of dealing with medical, social, and emotional issues. Only some of the suggestions may apply to you; of those, only some may be useful to you. Each of you entered the cancer experience a unique individual. Your treatment experience was unique, and so is your posttreatment situation. However, there are some near-universal issues for the cancer survivor that can be addressed.

This book assumes that you have achieved a complete remission (there is no evidence of remaining cancer) at the end of therapy. However, much of the information and advice applies as well if your cancer is stable on maintenance therapy or without therapy.

This book uses the word "family" to refer to those people who care for you. Your family may include children, parents, siblings, a spouse, a lover, close friends, or co-workers. The key is that these people care about you and are affected by your recovery.

You and your family can read this book cover to cover, using whatever information is helpful to you. Or you can skim the chapters for the questions that interest you now. Each section has bold-print questions followed by brief answers or outlines of how to get the answer.

Statements that reflect the book's philosophy or that can be used as mental tools or "handles" are highlighted in bold print. Repeated use of those handles that work well for you can make them progressively more effective. Handles that do not work well for you may prompt you to think of ones that do. The simplicity of handles makes them powerful when you are compromised by fear, anxiety, or fatigue, as well as when you are calm.

The appendixes include a glossary of basic terms, a selected annotated bibliography, a resource list for the patient who has completed cancer therapy, an explanation of the different types of health care workers, a guide for creating your personal medical records, a list of cancer's warning signs, steps for cancer prevention, and a summary of specific cancer screening.

As a cancer survivor, you are not so much ending a tumultuous journey as beginning a new phase of it. I hope to guide you through the months and years after completing your treatment, lessening the pain, loneliness, disappointment, and frustration that often accompany recovery. Use your experience with cancer as a catalyst to personal emotional and spiritual growth. There is life after cancer. Make it a good life.

Acknowledgments

I thank the following individuals who read the draft of *After Cancer* and offered input on the text: Marvin J. Stone, M.D., Lloyd Kitchens, M.D., Kristi J. McIntyre, M.D., Alan Brodsky, M.D., Rodger L. Bick, M.D., Julia H. Rowland, Ph.D., James P. Knochel, M.D., James F. Strauss, M.D., Monique Kunkel, M.D., Harold T. Vanderpool, Ph.D., Th.M., Pam Jenkins, M.S., Brenda S. Casey, R.N., O.C.N., Jill Guidrey, R.N., Becky O'Shea, M.S., R.N., O.C.N., Susan O'Steen Allen, Clare Chaney, Mimi Dimaio, Harriet Gross, Edward J. Harpham, Ellen Hermanson, Adele Hess, Larry G. Moore, Jessica Miller, Lisa Kessler, Deborah Rubin, M.A., Margaret C. Sheperd, Penny Ventura, and Sharon Witherspoon. Thanks also to Nancy Taylor for helping with my computer searches.

This book is comprehensive because other people shared their journeys with me through Dialogue, a support group for cancer survivors at Presbyterian Hospital of Dallas. I thank these people, who, through trust, caring, and mutual support, helped me understand many of the issues I and other cancer survivors faced. It was at Dialogue that I received many tools for coping with recovery and overcoming obstacles to healthy survivorship.

I am thankful to my primary doctors James Strauss, M.D., and

Susan Creagan, M.D., for their excellent and sensitive care during my journey through and after cancer. Physicians like Jim and Susan make me proud to be a part of our noble profession. I thank my gastroenterologist, Peter M. Loeb, M.D., my otolaryngologist, Roger Skiles, M.D., and my allergist, Gary N. Gross, M.D., for their skillful probing with both words and scopes. Thanks also to Paul Ellenbogen, M.D., radiologist, who has captured the pictures of my journey and who has delivered the news—good and bad—with care. Additional thanks to David G. Maloney, M.D., Ph.D., and Tina Marie Liles, R.N., of Stanford. They prove that clinical research is about the care of individual patients.

A special thanks to Pam Jenkins, oncology social worker, for her therapeutic listening and guidance. Every cancer survivor should have a Pam. I thank my rabbi, Jeffrey Leynor, who has prayed with and for me. He has helped me find and trust answers to difficult questions. I would also like to thank Pamela L. Sedwick, M.D., for her support and friendship. Pam offered me an ideal opportunity to return to the practice of internal medicine.

Cancer often allows people to discover a new dimension in old friends and to find new friends. Debra Sue Bruck, my older sister, became one of my closest friends through my cancer. Pam Krauss, my best friend since ninth grade, continues to listen, care, and offer advice with a constancy unmoved by changing circumstances. Cancer introduced me to two new friends, Susan O'Steen Allen and Sharon E. Witherspoon. Despite innumerable interruptions by our collective nine children between the ages of two weeks and seven years, we supported each other and learned together how to deal with cancer while raising these precious young people.

I appreciate the love and support provided by my parents, Joseph and Naomi Schlessel, and my parents-in-law, John and Jean Harpham. I also appreciate the continued concern and support of our extended families and friends.

I am grateful to Mary Cunnane, my editor at W. W. Norton, who shares my goal of helping others through books, and to Otto Sonntag, who polished the final draft with his artful copyediting.

This book owes much to my children, Rebecca, Jessica, and

William. Looking for healthy answers to their questions and fears encouraged me to find healthy answers for myself and others.

This book would not have been possible without the love and support of my husband, Ted. Together, we have walked and talked through all stages of our cancer experience and the writing of this book. He encouraged the writing of *After Cancer,* even when it meant pizza for dinner (again) and keeping the kids occupied while I finished "one last page."

AFTER CANCER

—

A GUIDE TO YOUR NEW LIFE

1

Understanding the Medical Aspects of Recovery

Most of you would like to put your whole cancer experience completely behind you. You would like to say, "I had cancer, but it's all over now. I am, or soon will be, as healthy as I was before I got sick. I can go back to my routine medical care."

Can you really face your future by ignoring your history of cancer? Should you? Unless your doctors have given you a 100 percent guarantee that your cancer will never come back, you will have some concern about recurrent cancer. Depending on what treatment you received, your body will need to recuperate. And many treatments cause their own problems, in the short run or the long run.

Your health is not the same as it was before you developed cancer. Your knowledge about the vulnerability of your health is painfully changed. Believing that you are back to the way you were before cancer may save you immediate anxiety about possible future problems. But it would be at an enormous cost to you, emotionally and physically.

There are many reasons why you should continue learning about your cancer. In the short run, you can take steps to prevent or minimize problems, and thus maximize and speed your recovery. In the long run, knowledge allows you to take measures to help prevent future problems such as recurrent cancer (recurrence) or the development of a new type of cancer.

You have met the challenge of treatments. But your situation is like that of a marathon runner, whose efforts are not over at the end of the race. Successful runners are careful about their recovery. For days afterward they get extra fluids, nutrients, and rest. They know that it takes weeks to get their primed, but spent, bodies completely back to normal.

Given that an optimally conditioned runner has to make adjustments to recover from a race, imagine the needs of a competitive runner who sprains her ankle. She has to decide how to deal with her injury. She can ignore the injury and risk further injury while performing at less than peak performance. Or she can find out what to do to maximize and speed her recovery. This may mean slowing down or even stopping her training schedule for a while. If, after complete healing, some ankle weakness remains, she can act as if there were no problem, running in pain and risking recurrent injury. Or she can learn about modifications to make in her shoes, running style, training schedule, or running route that would allow continued, though changed, running.

Your cancer and treatment caused changes in your body that can take days, weeks, months, or even years to disappear. Some changes may be permanent. Like the runner, you will feel better and heal faster if you learn about the changes in your body and the ways to help yourself recover.

Many survivors who have completed treatment struggle with a sense of vulnerability and an urgent desire to do something to help protect their renewed health. Learning what you can do to stay healthy will allow you to regain a sense of control and will maximize your chance of staying healthy.

After cancer, you may feel bombarded by information about what causes, cures, or prevents cancer. Newspapers and magazines, books, and well-meaning friends and family offer frightening, exciting, confusing, and often contradictory messages. Knowledge can help you sort out useful facts from inaccurate or misleading stories.

Each year brings advances in the diagnosis and treatment of

cancer. In the future, new options for screening, follow-up, and preventive measures for your type of cancer may be offered to you. Staying informed about your medical situation after cancer will make it easier for you to appreciate the benefits of these developments.

This chapter will help you to understand what is happening medically after your treatment is complete and to participate in your own care. It reviews the medicine of reevaluation, recovery, and long-term care after cancer. The text assumes that you have a working knowledge of the basics of cancer medicine as it applies to a newly diagnosed cancer patient. "Diagnosis," "prognosis," "staging," "biopsy," and "scan" are all terms covered in *Diagnosis: Cancer: Your Guide through the First Few Months.*

REEVALUATION

What Happens Now That My Cancer Treatment Is Completed?

Completing cancer treatment thrusts you into a new phase of dealing with your cancer. This is a time of crucial information gathering and decision making. You will

- find out the status of your cancer. Is your cancer completely gone as far as we can tell? If your cancer is not gone, where is it?
- evaluate your current condition (your physical and emotional limits, both temporary and permanent). How are your kidneys? Lungs? Heart? Weight?
- make a decision about whether further treatment will offer any benefit in terms of maximizing control of your cancer now or decreasing the chance of its coming back
- begin to learn how to live most fully within any new limits
- learn what you can do to accelerate your recovery
- find out what you can do to prevent future problems, such as use sunscreen or undergo periodic colon tests
- begin the adjustment of changing from being a patient under active cancer treatment to being a patient with a history of can-

cer who is seen for checkups geared to the special needs of someone who survived your type of cancer
- begin your lifelong routine of cancer follow-up

What Is Restaging?

Restaging is the evaluation after your treatment is completed, to determine

- how much cancer is left, if any
- whether there are any new areas of cancer

How Is Restaging Done?

Your restaging is orchestrated by your oncologist, who will

- talk to you about any symptoms or problems you are having
- examine you ("do a physical exam")
- order various tests and studies, such as blood tests, X rays, and scans, or bone marrow biopsies

Sometimes surgery is advised as part of your restaging. This may be expected, such as "second-look" surgeries for certain types of ovarian cancer. Or you may need surgery because there is still something on your scan or your exam, and because there is no other way to determine whether it is cancer or a scar. As blood tests and imaging studies become more and more sophisticated, surgery is used less frequently for restaging.

Why Is Restaging Important?

Restaging allows your doctors to

- evaluate your response to the treatments
- determine whether further treatment is indicated
- redetermine your prognosis

Will My Restaging Comprise All of the Same Tests as My Original Staging?

The tests used to restage you will depend on the type of cancer you had, which tests were abnormal when you were first diagnosed, and what new tests have become available since then. In many cases all the tests that were done when you were first diagnosed will be repeated. Sometimes fewer tests are needed. Rarely, more tests are needed.

When Should I Be Restaged?

Most cancer treatments continue to have effects on cancer cells for a while after the last treatment is administered. Therefore, restaging is undertaken when your treatment has had ample time to have its maximum effect.

How Long after I Receive My Last Cancer Treatment Will the Treatment Kill Cancer Cells (Have an Antitumor Effect)?

Depending on what kind of cancer you had, and what kind of therapy you had, your treatments can continue to have an effect on cancer cells for weeks to months. This activity against cancer cells is the "antitumor effect."

Surgery itself has no further effect on your cancer once the operation is complete. However, the physical changes that accompany removing a cancer from the body and healing from the surgery may have an antitumor effect in some people. There is reason to believe that for some people the stimulation of the immune system during the healing process after surgery may also have an antitumor effect.

Chemotherapy continues to work for days to weeks after the drug is given. That is one of the reasons why the doses are spaced out over time.

Radiation therapy continues to have an antitumor effect for weeks after the last dose is given.

Immunotherapy continues to work over days to weeks—and

possibly months to years, if it causes a self-perpetuating change in your immune system.

The exact duration of the antitumor effect is not predictable, but it can be estimated on the basis of

- the type of cancer
- the type of therapy
- the presence of concurrent therapy
- the duration and intensity of cancer therapy
- your body's response to the cancer therapy
- your nutritional and circulation status

Do I Really Need to Have All of These Tests?

These tests are needed to determine whether you have received enough treatment and to be sure that no new problems are developing. Getting accurate information and making good decisions *after* treatment is just as important as doing so before treatment, as far as your long-term health goes.

What about the Risk to Me from Getting All These Scans and X Rays?

Your recent cancer poses a clear and present danger to your health. Making the best treatment decisions on the basis of complete and accurate information is critical to maximizing your health. Your risks from the X-ray exposure are far less than the risks of not evaluating adequately your cancer situation.

X rays should not be taken indiscriminately. You can minimize your exposure to X rays when there are acceptable alternative ways of getting the *same* information, such as sonograms. When you have doubts about the necessity of an X ray, ask your doctor

- what information will be obtained from the X ray
- how the information gained will affect your decision making
- whether you can get the same information without X rays

What Is My Prognosis after Treatment?

Your prognosis is the statistical prediction of how you will do. Your overall prognosis is your long-term chance of survival.

Many types of cancer have a good short-term prognosis but a poor long-term prognosis. For example, your cancer may be incurable with current forms of therapy, but is so slow growing that you are expected to survive for many years. Or your type of cancer may be expected to respond well to initial treatments, but has a high rate of recurrence and loses this responsiveness.

Prognosis may be described in general statements such as "Your prognosis is very good" or "Your prognosis is poor." Oftentimes, when you want to hear something more specific, you will be given a percentage, such as "Your prognosis for a five-year survival is 60 percent."

To say that you have a 60 percent chance of staying in remission for at least five years means that for every 100 persons with your type of cancer who received your type of treatment and achieved remission, 60 will stay in remission for at least five years and 40 will develop recurrent cancer. In five years each individual patient will either be in 100 percent remission or have a recurrence.

To say that you have a 60 percent chance of surviving for at least five years means that for every 100 persons in your situation, 60 will be alive in five years. Some of those 60 will be disease-free, some will have had recurrent disease and be back in remission, and some will be living with active cancer.

Your prognosis after treatment may be different from that when you were first diagnosed. This is because your doctors have two important pieces of information unavailable before you were treated: they know whether your cancer responds to treatment, and they know how healthy you are after treatment.

For illustration, let us say that when you were originally diagnosed, you were told that you had a 50 percent chance of surviving at least five years. If you did well with treatment, you may now be told that you have a 95 percent chance of surviving at least five years. This improvement in your chance of survival has occurred because the original figure of 50 percent included those people who would not respond to the therapy as well as those who would die of complications before achieving remission. At the time of your diagnosis, doctors knew your *chance* of responding, but could not know how your cancer would in fact respond. The figure of 95 percent given to you after your treatment is derived from information showing that, of the people who did as well as you did, 95 percent were alive five years later.

One thing to keep in mind is that your prognosis keeps changing as your situation changes. The prognosis given to you when you were first diagnosed is not as relevant or meaningful as the prognosis based on your current situation.

Factors that help determine your prognosis include

- your type of cancer
- the stage of your cancer at the time you were diagnosed
- your cancer's response to treatments
- your level of physical fitness
- the presence or absence of other medical conditions
- available indicators specific for your type of cancer, such as tumor markers and hormone receptors
- many factors that we cannot measure, such as your "will to live"

How Reliable Is My Prognosis?

Your prognosis does not tell you how you as an individual will do. It is a statistical probability that helps predict patterns of outcome in populations of people with your illness. Many people with a 2 percent chance of cure at the time they were diagnosed are now cured of their cancer; conversely, many people who had a 95 percent chance of cure at the time they were diagnosed succumbed to their cancer. There is no way to predict which individuals will be on the unfortunate side of great statistics and which on the exceptionally good side of terrible statistics. Favorable statistics do not guarantee that you will do well; unfavorable statistics do not guarantee that you will do poorly. Some individuals have recovered from every type of cancer; every type of cancer can be treated in some way.

Statistics say nothing about how you as an individual will do.

If My Prognosis Tells Me Nothing Definite about How I Will Do, Why Am I Ever Told My Prognosis?

Your prognosis is useful when it is considered to be one of many factors that help you and your doctors decide when and how to treat your cancer. It is also important in helping you make major decisions, such as those involved in family, career, and financial planning.

It must be emphasized that your prognosis does not guarantee anything one way or the other. One man was given a poor prognosis. After he started chemotherapy, he broke off his marriage engagement, dropped out of the amateur baseball league that he loved, and settled into a routine of going to work and then coming home to "wait for the end." His cancer responded, and he remained in remission ten years later. During those ten years, his fiancée moved away and married, and his baseball team won three pennants. His prognosis may have been bad, but he did well.

The unreliability of your prognosis can misguide you the opposite way, too. One woman was told that her prognosis was excellent, with a 96 percent chance of cure. Encouraged, she proceeded with her lifelong plans to start her own business. Unfortunately, she was one of the 4 percent who were not cured. She became too ill to work and lost all her savings in her business before it had a chance to succeed. Statistically speaking, she may have had a greater chance of being killed in a car accident than of having a recurrence, so her decision to proceed with the business was very reasonable. The point is that your prognosis provides no guarantee as to what happens with your cancer.

What Is Maintenance Therapy?

Some cancers are not curable but can be held in check with maintenance therapy. This usually consists of lower-dose medication taken indefinitely that

• slows down or stops the growth of the cancer
• is fairly well tolerated

The goals of maintenance therapy are to

• preserve a disease-free state (help prevent recurrence) after remission is achieved
• help prevent progression of persistent cancer when curative therapy is not available
• help prevent progression of persistent cancer and minimize complications from persistent cancer when curative therapy is too risky
• buy time while waiting for more effective or less toxic therapy
• promote physical and psychological comfort

What Is Remission?

Remission is the absence of any detectable sign of your cancer after restaging tests are completed. "Remission" is used synonymously with "complete remission."

Remission is not the same as cure. Your remission can last for one month, one year, one decade, or the rest of your life. You must remain in complete remission for a length of time specific for your type of cancer to be considered cured. Many people achieve complete remission but are not cured.

What Is a Durable Remission?

A durable remission is one that lasts for a long time. How long "long" is depends on the usual expectations for your type of cancer and is a subjective notion. A durable remission is not the same as a cure.

For example, if you have a type of cancer that usually recurs within five years of achieving remission and you have been in remission for eight years, you are deemed to have a durable remission. If your type of cancer usually recurs within one year of remission and you enjoy three years of remission, this is felt to represent a durable remission.

If My X Ray or Scan Still Has Spots on It, or Some of My Blood Tests Are Not Normal, How Can the Doctors Say I Am in Remission?

It is very possible for your X rays, scans, or blood tests to remain abnormal even though no evidence of cancer is detected. X rays and scans can remain abnormal because the treatments got rid of all the cancer cells but left a scar in the area. This situation is similar to that of a skin infection that is cured with antibiotics but heals with a permanent visible scar, or that of a pneumonia that resolves but leaves a permanent spot on your chest X ray. Blood tests can remain abnormal, reflecting the changes that occur as your body recovers from the treatment.

How Do Doctors Know Which Spots Are Cancer and Which Are Scars?

Your doctors can usually know whether a spot on an X ray or scan represents a scar or leftover cancer on the basis of

- subtle differences between the appearances of scars and cancer
- the different behaviors over time of scars and cancer

When there is any doubt, and the answer will affect decisions that need to be made at this time, the only way to be sure whether a spot is cancer is to biopsy the spot.

How Do Doctors Know Whether an Abnormal Result on a Blood Test Is Due to Cancer?

Your blood test results are interpreted with regard to all the other available information about your specific circumstances. For example, if you develop elevated liver enzymes in your blood, this does not suggest cancer if your type of cancer rarely spreads to the liver and if your treatment is expected to cause such an elevation.

Sometimes your blood tests will indicate abnormalities that cannot be explained completely. If the results of your physical exam and various scans do not explain the abnormality, your doctor may have to watch and wait to determine the significance of the blood test abnormality.

It is not uncommon to have unexplained abnormalities that persist for a while, or indefinitely, following cancer treatment. These abnormalities often have no impact on people's lives or their prognoses. The surviving of cancer may mean living with "blips and spots" on tests.

What Is a Response or a Partial Remission?

You have had a response, also called a partial remission, when tests indicate that you still have cancer but that you have gotten rid of at least half of your cancer. This can be determined through a comparison of the results of tests obtained before and after treatment. For example, the spots on your chest X ray may be 75 percent smaller (e.g., in lung cancer), or there may be 75 percent fewer cancer cells in the blood and bone marrow (e.g., in leukemia). Some doctors may use the term "response" or "partial remission" when there is *any* shrinkage of your cancer, but a less than 50 percent reduction in detectable cancer is not considered a meaningful improvement from an overall view of your cancer situation. Ask your doctors what they mean when they use the terms "response" and "partial remission."

What Is a Cure?

A cure is said to have occurred when there is no detectable sign of cancer and you have the same life expectancy as if you had never had cancer. For some cancers you have to be in complete remission for a year to be considered cured. For many others five years is the reliable interval after which your chance of recurrence is extremely low. Still others, such as certain types of lymphoma, are considered incurable, because no matter how long you live in complete remission there is still a significant chance the cancer will recur.

Do I Have to Be Told I Am "Cured" of My Cancer in Order to Hope to Feel Normal Again?

Absolutely not. Normal life after any crisis or change means learning how to adjust to all the changes. You will probably not feel the same after surviving cancer as you did before your diagnosis, but you can feel normal again.

Change, loss, and fear are not unique to cancer survivors. Many chronic diseases other than cancer require ongoing medical care and demand changes in the day-to-day details of diet, activities, and relationships. Survivors of other chronic diseases work, lead stable family lives, and feel normal. People with diabetes, arthritis, or emphysema learn to adjust and compensate for their physical problems with the help of medications, physical therapy, walking aids, and dietary restrictions. Each of these diseases is potentially life threatening, yet people learn to live well and feel normal again, despite the risks and limitations imposed by their illness. These people do not feel the same as they did before their illness began, but they feel normal. People living with cancer can learn to lead normal, fulfilled lives, too, despite the need for ongoing follow-up and therapy.

Feeling normal is a state of mind in which you are adjusted to your circumstances. Maintaining your sense of normal throughout life involves accepting and adjusting to an unending series of changes, whether related to aging, illness, or injury. You would have had to adjust to some physical changes even if you had not developed cancer.

Unwanted change is an issue for everyone. Healthy fifty-year-olds are very different physically, emotionally, and spiritually from their earlier, adolescent selves. Yet a healthy fifty-year-old person usually feels "normal" despite the changes in vision, hair and body fat distribution, and muscle mass. Many of the changes accompanying cancer resemble those of healthy aging. There is much to be learned from people who grow old gracefully and continue to live full lives throughout their days.

You may resent or resist having to make adjustments after completing your cancer therapy. Understandably, it is easier to adjust to age-related than to cancer-related changes, because they are gradual, expected, and shared by others in your age group. With time, you can adjust to the unexpected, relatively sudden changes brought on by your cancer and its treatment. Normal life, with or without cancer, involves change.

Another reality needs to be mentioned: being in remission long enough to be considered "cured" does not magically eliminate the fears, anxieties, and potential medical problems. Too many people who are cured of their cancer continue to have medical or emotional problems related to their earlier treatment. Being cured does not necessarily make you feel normal.

Whether or not you feel normal or happy depends on how you adjust to the changes related to your cancer. Many survivors in temporary remission from incurable cancers or with stable, persistent cancer, as well as those who are cured, experience fulfilling, happy, normal lives without significant physical or emotional problems.

Take steps both to maximize the meaning and enjoyment of each day and to maximize your chance for cure or durable remission. Working toward the goal of personal peace and fulfillment is life enriching, and possibly life lengthening, no matter what your circumstances.

Cure is not a magical state where all problems end. Aim for personal peace no matter what the specifics of your cancer situation.

Do I Need a Second Opinion after I Complete My Therapy?

To get a second opinion, you go to a different doctor who, after reviewing your case, gives you his or her opinion of your situation and advises you about treatment. Most people seek a second opinion when they are first diagnosed, before treatment is begun. In many circumstances a second opinion is also valuable after completion of treatment. For example, it is useful if

• you did not obtain one before you were treated, or
• there are multiple treatment options for your cancer, or

- there are multiple options regarding further treatment after remission is achieved, or
- you are unsure of your current status or the options available to you at this time, or
- you have persistent cancer after treatment is completed, or
- you want a second opinion about your reevaluation or your future follow-up

A second opinion is probably unnecessary if

- you did well with your treatments, and
- you are confident about your reevaluation, your understanding of all the options available to you at this time for further treatment, follow-up of your cancer, and prevention of future problems, and
- you do not feel the need for a second opinion

A second opinion allows you to review all your current options and confirm current decisions. It provides needed reassurance and lets you feel more confident about these important decisions.

You rely on additional opinions for many other decisions. For example, most of you read *Consumer Reports,* talk with friends, and do some comparative shopping before buying a car. Or if a mechanic told you that you needed an $800 part to fix the "clank" in your car, you would probably get a second opinion before agreeing to the repair (unless you were a car mechanic yourself). Your health is obviously more valuable than your car.

Are There Downsides to Getting a Second Opinion?

Gathering and sorting information, and trying to make life-and-death decisions, is an emotionally draining process that consumes enormous amounts of time and energy. Your reserves are depleted at the end of treatment. Wanting to avoid stress, you may be tempted to hurry the closure of your cancer experience. Rest assured that the short-term disadvantages of directing energies to getting a second opinion are far outweighed by the benefits of an informed decision about further treatment and follow-up.

When you go for a second opinion, the new doctor will perhaps inform you that he or she would have advised different treatment for your cancer when you were first diagnosed. Obviously, this does not help you in any way, since you can never go back to where you were and make the decision again. Even though it is just one doctor's opinion, knowing that you might have been treated differently can make you feel anxious about something that you cannot change.

A more common problem is that you will receive conflicting information or advice about your current situation. You will have to sort out which information to believe and which advice to follow. This process of deciding what to do with conflicting advice can be extremely stressful. In the long run, however, gathering information and sorting through the options will provide you the lifelong comfort of knowing that you made decisions on the basis of the best information available at the time.

Weigh and balance the answers to the following questions, and you will get an idea of the best option for you:

- What are all the treatment options available to me now, both conventional and investigational?
- What is the cure rate of each option?
- What is the response rate of each option?
- What are the short-term risks of each option?
- What are the long-term risks of each option?
- What are the risks of a second cancer?
- What are the risks of future medical problems?
- Will any current treatment options limit future treatment options?

How Do I Decide What to Do If the Oncologist Providing the Second Opinion Disagrees with My Original Oncologist?

Oftentimes, when doctors do not agree on how to manage your situation, it is because no single "best" treatment exists. When treatments are fairly new, definitive answers about long-term risks and benefits may not be available. Each doctor's conclusions and advice regarding your situation are based on many factors, such as his or her

- clinical experience (the successes and failures seen personally with various treatments)
- involvement in clinical research
- interpretation of the available data (different doctors can draw different conclusions from the same data)

The treatments being used most often in their medical center or locale (standard of care for the community) may also affect doctors' approaches.

If you get conflicting advice, have each oncologist explain his or her advice in light of the controversy. You can determine how simple or elaborate an explanation you want or need (you do not have to learn everything about car repair to make a decision about which mechanic to use). After sorting through the various recommendations, you will feel either that there is one "best" choice or that there is more than one "right" choice.

For example, you may be in remission and your doctor feels that you have had enough treatment. If you pursue a second opinion, another oncologist may recommend an extra two months of chemotherapy "just to be safe." Much as you would like to be done with treatment, you want to do what is best in the long run.

One possible outcome of this scenario is that you weigh the risks and benefits of each option as explained by both doctors, and proceed with the original advice. You will feel more confident about the decision to stop treatments, because you looked at your options. Consider the similar case of people buying a house who fall in love with the first one they see. The school district, floor plan, and price seem perfect. The house "feels right," down to the telephone outlets. Still, most people would check out other houses on the market to reinforce their impression. If they find an even better house, one that "*really* feels right," they will be happy that they did not sign a contract on the first house. If they come back to buy the first, they will feel surer of the decision.

Getting a second opinion and working through your options at the completion of your treatments will make you feel more comfortable when, later, you read or hear about other patients with your type of cancer who pursued one of the other treatment options. You will be more relaxed, knowing that you investigated and rejected those options as not the best for you.

Another outcome could be that the doctors providing the conflicting advice discuss the situation, after which they come to one recommendation. Or they may conclude that your options are equally good, in which case other factors (preferred doctor, treatment location, financial concerns, etc.) will determine your final decision. When there are a number of right ways to treat you, you will feel that this resolution of conflicting opinions steered you to the best treatment for you.

The most stressful outcome is that the doctors continue to disagree after discussion with you and with each other. Whom do you believe? How do you decide what is best to do? Additional second opinions (third and fourth opinions) may resolve the conflict. How you feel (your intuition) may help guide you to the best treatment choice for you. Discussing the situation with your internist may help. Usually you will end up proceeding with one option as the best of a number of options. Since not everyone can be right, you may have to dismiss the advice of one or more of the doctors in order to proceed.

There are always options at each phase of your journey with cancer. Knowledge of your options allows you to make the best choice for you with the information available.

Will My Oncologist Feel Upset If I Go for a Second Opinion?

Your doctor wants you to do well physically and emotionally. Doctors expect people to get second and third opinions when people feel the need. Doctors are professionals whose work routinely involves getting and giving second opinions.

You may feel more concerned about your doctor's feelings when you go for a second opinion after completing treatment than after your original diagnosis. After all, your doctor has invested time, energy, and emotions to help get you where you are. You do not want your actions to be interpreted as an expression of lack of satisfaction or trust.

Second opinions are part of cancer survivorship. You have a right to be as sure as possible about decisions that affect your life.

If you sense disapproval on the part of your doctor for your desiring a second opinion, step back and see whether you are perhaps interpreting your self-consciousness as your doctor's disapproval. If you are sure that your doctor is unhappy about your getting another opinion, consider switching doctors. It is a red flag when your doctor urges you not to get a second opinion or threatens to stop caring for you if you do. This is an especially difficult situation if you live in a small town with only one or two available oncologists.

If you find yourself going from doctor to doctor, never feeling satisfied with the advice you are receiving, get professional counseling to help you learn how to assess your options and make decisions about your care.

FOLLOW-UP

You are a cancer survivor. Although you would like to put your cancer totally behind you, you are different now. In order to minimize your chance of future problems, you need to be evaluated periodically for evidence of problems from your cancer or its treatment. This section will teach you about your follow-ups and about available treatments aimed at keeping you healthy and preventing recurrence.

What Is the Purpose of Routine Follow-up?

Regularly scheduled checkups allow your oncologist to "follow you." This involves

- monitoring the continuing response to your treatments
- evaluating and treating problems left over from your cancer or cancer treatments
- looking for signs of complications or aftereffects of the treatments
- looking for signs of recurrent cancer

What Determines What Is Needed at My Follow-up Visits and Their Frequency?

Many factors affect the specifics of your follow-up evaluations:

- your type of cancer
- your type of treatment
- the length of time since your last treatment
- the stage of your cancer at the time of diagnosis
- the rapidity with which your cancer was growing at the time of diagnosis
- the presence or absence of persistent problems related to your cancer or cancer therapy (e.g., abnormal blood tests and lung/ digestive/kidney problems)
- tests needed for data collection if you were part of a clinical trial

The routine follow-up schedule provides only a broad guideline. Exactly when you have your follow-up and what is done there must be tailored to your circumstances.

Do I Wait for My Follow-up to Ask Questions or Report New Problems?

Routine exams are scheduled with the presumption that you have no new symptoms or problems, in the hope of picking up problems before you develop any symptoms. You should not wait for a routine follow-up if you have a new problem. A woman underwent a mastectomy for breast cancer six years ago. She faithfully went for her biannual cancer follow-ups, seeing them as her safety net to keep her healthy. At her recent checkup, she reported a small lump in her remaining breast that she had noticed two months earlier. She had not called the doctor, because she knew that it could be taken care of at her routine checkup. Her misunderstanding of her role in her follow-ups caused a two-month delay in the diagnosis and treatment of her new cancer. Your doctor cannot call you every week to check on you; he or she depends on you to report promptly any changes.

Your doctor can tell you the plan for your follow-up schedule. For example, you may be scheduled for checkups with your doctor every three months and scans every six months for the first year, then for checkups every six months and scans every twelve months for the next two years, and then for annual checkups and scans. This rough schedule will be adapted to your individual needs. If you have ongoing medical problems, or if you develop new ones, you will need to be seen more often than is usual for a posttreatment patient.

Your doctor can tailor your follow-up to your circumstances only if you keep him or her informed of your progress, problems, and questions. When you develop new problems between checkups, notify your doctor or nurse so that the timing of your next visit can be moved up if necessary.

You play a key role in optimizing the timing and efficiency of your follow-up by keeping your doctor well informed of your condition.

Get a list of signs and symptoms about which your oncologist wants to be notified right away. If you develop something not on your list and if you are uncertain about whether you should call, call your doctor's office and ask whether you should

- wait for your scheduled appointment to discuss the question or problem
- talk to the doctor on the telephone
- come in earlier than your scheduled appointment to see the doctor

When in doubt about calling your doctor, call. It is better to sound a false alarm than to have a treatable problem get out of control or cause unnecessary discomfort or anxiety. You owe it to yourself and your family not to take chances.

What Can I Expect at My Routine Follow-ups?

Generally speaking, all routine follow-up visits will include your doctor's talking to you about any changes since your last visit (taking a history) and examining you (performing a physical exam). The physical exam may be very brief or very thorough, depending on the type of cancer you had and how you are doing. Routine exams often include blood tests and sometimes an X ray.

Some of your follow-up visits, such as your "one year after completion of treatment" checkup, will entail a complete reevaluation. These comprehensive checkups usually include a thorough history and exam, as well as more extensive testing (blood tests, X rays, scans).

At the end of each visit, your doctor will review his or her conclusions about how you are doing, and any plans regarding future follow-up and treatment.

What Do I Need to Know about My Follow-up?

In order to optimize the benefit and efficiency of your follow-up visits, know

- the proposed schedule of visits
- the proposed schedule of tests
- the purpose of each visit (some visits will be quick rechecks and others will be comprehensive reevaluations)
- whether you should fast (not eat or drink anything) before the visit (many times you are allowed water or black coffee when fasting)
- whether you need to do anything special about your medicines just prior to your visit (some medicines, such as diabetes pills, should not be taken when you are fasting; some may interfere with your tests)

Do I Have to Prepare for My Follow-up Visits?

Patients often complain that doctors focus right away on the physical problems, ask countless questions, and never have enough time for explanations or for just a normal conversation. Many patients recoil at the idea of preparing a list of questions and problems, feeling that they should not be treated like a car being brought to the shop. Or they worry that a list would make them look like a hypochondriac. Patients understandably want to feel that they are being treated like a whole person.

The purpose of each follow-up visit is for you to get your needs taken care of and for the doctor to be certain that everything is being done to ensure that you do as well as possible. In order for you to receive the best care, you and your doctor must work together as a team. Your job is to describe your problems and explain your concerns as clearly as possible. Most people do this best with some advance preparation.

Like everyone else, doctors face time constraints. What you may interpret as abruptness may be your doctor's attempt to be organized, so that the information obtained is complete and accurate and so that your most serious problems are addressed. A vague, unstructured discussion or a focus on one issue may make you feel better emotionally but divert your doctor from the important issues.

Your oncologist is trying to understand your medical situation, find the best solutions to your medical problems, and prevent new problems from occurring. Most oncologists truly care as much about your emotional well-being as about your physical well-being, but focus primarily on the physical in order to maximize the chance that you are physically well enough to deal with the emotional. From a practical viewpoint your doctors are the only people who can address the major medical issues (as opposed to nurses, social workers, counselors, and so on). If they do not take care of these questions and problems, no one else can. Also, if oncologists did not maintain some distance and objectivity, they could not make the best medical decisions for you.

At the beginning of each of your visits, you are like a mystery person. Even if your doctor has been taking care of you for years, he or she has to figure out what your problems and concerns are that day in order to address them. And, as with any mystery, the more clues you provide, the faster and more accurate will be your doctor's solutions.

If you just show up for your visit and expect to sort through your problems and questions while your doctor listens, or if you expect your doctor to figure out your problems and questions through doctor-directed questions, you may spend most of the visit just figuring out what your problems are.

It is much easier for everyone if you tell your doctor, "I have had some cramping in my stomach and have noticed some blood in my bowel movements for the past three weeks," than if the doctor has to keep prodding: "Are there any problems?" "Yes." "Can you tell me what the problem is?" "My bowel movements are different." "How are they different?" "I think there has been some blood in them." "When did this begin?" "Let me see . . . today is June 12, so it must have been two . . . no wait, it was about three weeks ago." "Do you have any pain?" "Yes." And so on.

There is an old joke about the patient in the emergency room who complains of stomach pain and vomits blood. After the usual series of questions and physical examinations, the emergency room doctor orders an X ray, which shows a razor blade in the stomach, and asks the patient, "Why didn't you tell me that you swallowed a razor blade?" The patient answers, "Because you didn't ask me!"

You are not expected to be an expert at describing your symptoms and problems, but it will be less stressful for you if you are prepared to discuss your problems and concerns. You will be better served, too, because the information you provide will be more accurate and more complete. How many times have you left the doctor's office and realized that you forgot to mention something important?

Your emotional, social, and spiritual concerns and problems are just as important as your medical ones. Your oncologist absolutely needs to be aware of cancer-related sexual difficulties, problems with your children, problems with insurance or your job, and the like. By making your doctor aware of these issues, he or she can better understand your condition, better understand you, and direct you to appropriate people who can help you deal with your problems.

It does not make sense, however, for your oncologist to be counseling you at length, trying to resolve these issues. It is in your best interests if your oncologist directs you to the people who can help you.

Ironically, the more focused and direct the exchange of information at the beginning of your visit, the more time and energy is left to discuss your emotional and social concerns, to relate socially as two people, and for your doctor to offer comfort and support.

You are a person, with feelings and a soul. When you go to your doctor, you are not taking your body to the shop; you are trusting your being to another person. Your doctor can best care for you through a team effort at understanding and solving your problems.

How Can I Prepare for My Doctor Visits?

Before your visit, rank your concerns and questions in order of importance to you. Do not leave anything out, because what you consider minor or insignificant may turn out to be a critical piece of information to your doctor.

Think about how to present your information in a concise yet complete way. You may find that it helps to compose a list to bring to your visit. If there is not enough time to cover everything at your visit, the prepared list will help ensure that you cover the issues most important to you. Your doctor can glance at the list and spot any potential serious problems that must be addressed.

Before your visit

- make a list of any physical and emotional problems you have been experiencing
- make a list of your questions about your condition, your problems, your evaluation, your treatments
- know what time you need to be there
- know whether you need to be fasting

Every doctor has an individual style. Some doctors may appreciate your coming prepared with a list; others may be put off. The list is for you, so that you can keep your thoughts organized. Find ways to make your visits efficient and satisfying.

It helps to have a friend or family member accompany you. Even at routine follow-up visits, you may not remember everything your doctor says. Having a second listener takes some of the pressure off of you at the visit. You may appreciate reviewing and discussing the visit with your companion immediately afterward.

Am I Supposed to Tell My Doctor about Every Little Ache or Noticeable Change?

It is very common to be self-conscious about what you report at your checkups. Report anything that

- you suspect might be important
- a family member suspects might be important
- is keeping you from feeling well

If you are unsure whether something is important enough to bring up, err on the side of overreporting. Let your doctor decide what needs to be pursued. Attending to relatively minor comfort issues can make an enormous impact on the speed or comfort of your recovery.

Your doctor can help you only with things about which you tell him or her. Your doctor wants to save your life *and* take care of all your discomforts and worries.

Are There Any Options in Regard to My Follow-up?

Yes. Your doctor will advise a certain schedule of follow-up. If you have special needs, let your doctor know so that these needs can be factored in when planning your follow-up. Rest assured that your doctor is going to make your health, not your preferences or special needs, the overriding concern when arranging the details of your follow-up. Special needs that might affect timing of follow-up include

- travel restrictions (if you come in from out of town, some dates may be more expensive or less convenient than others)
- financial constraints (sometimes there is an option about how often certain tests are obtained or which tests are done)
- family/work responsibilities
- anxiety about your condition (for your peace of mind you may need more frequent follow-ups than are usually recommended)

Some patients prefer to have all their tests done prior to the follow-up visit, so that all the results can be discussed at the visit.

Where you are followed up can be influenced by travel restrictions or financial constraints. If your oncologist is in another city or town, you can sometimes arrange to have blood tests or scans performed locally, and the results or scans mailed to your oncologist. When very specialized blood tests are required that are not available locally, blood can sometimes be drawn locally and mailed to the lab used by your oncologist.

Follow-up visits help you stay well and confirm that you are doing well. Follow-ups do not cause cancer or other medical problems. Learn to use your follow-ups in a positive way.

Am I at Increased Risk for Noncancer Medical Problems?

You may be at increased risk for a variety of medical problems. Some of these involve changes that are seen in most people as they get older but that occur earlier in people who have received certain cancer therapies. Other problems are very uncommon unless the person was exposed to certain cancer therapies in the past. Specific problems are discussed in Chapter 2.

If My Doctor Keeps Ordering Blood Tests, Why Do I Need So Many If I Am Doing Fine?

After treatment is completed, your body will continue to undergo changes related to

- healing
- aftereffects of the cancer
- aftereffects of the treatments
- development of new problems if new problems develop

Your body has an amazing capacity to compensate for small problems. You can feel and look normal even when something is not right in your body. Blood tests offer one easy, risk-free, relatively cheap way to get additional information that may indicate the presence of a small problem that, if left untreated, can become a big problem. Scans and X rays, in contrast, are much more expensive and carry some risks. It is not practical or wise to perform them too often.

Why Is It Important to Know for What Diseases and Problems I Am at Risk?

You may be thinking, "I don't want to know about all my risks or about all the potential problems I can have. I've been through enough already." Your risks exist whether you are aware of them or not.

Knowledge allows you to choose to decrease the chance of developing certain problems. You can minimize your risk of skin changes due to radiation by staying out of the sun and using a moisturizer regularly.

Knowledge enables you to decrease the potential impact of these problems on your overall health through aggressive screening and evaluation at the earliest sign of any problem. This is done at your cancer follow-ups and your routine visits with your internist or general practitioner. If you are at a high risk of developing low thyroid because of radiation to the thyroid area, dangerously low thyroid hormone levels can be completely avoided with regular (annual) blood tests of thyroid function and more frequent blood tests if you ever develop subtle symptoms that suggest low thyroid. This approach will not prevent you from developing low thyroid; it will prevent significant symptoms or problems from low thyroid. Your risks exist whether you are aware of them or not.

Finding out about potential problems can be distressing at first. But in the long run, knowledge is power. If you are aware of your risks, you can gain some control over their impact on your overall health.

Learning about your risks of future problems enhances your ability to make good decisions about your life.

If My Checkup and Blood Work Are Okay, Can I Be Sure I Have No Cancer?

No. There is a limit to what tests and scans show. A cancer can be too small to be detected with current techniques, or it can be in a place that escapes current methods of detection.

Your doctor will talk with you, examine you, and order appropriate tests to look for cancer. This approach allows doctors, with reasonable risk and cost to you, to pick up most detectable cancers.

What Is a Recurrence?

If you were in complete remission (no evidence of cancer) for any length of time and now there is evidence that the same cancer has come back, you have had a recurrence of your cancer. The returning cancer is called a recurrence.

Each cancer is defined by the organ in which it originated, the organ in which the first cell became cancerous. Your cancer can recur in a different place from where it appeared earlier or in the same place. It has to be the same kind of cancer to be a recurrence. If you had prostate cancer confined to the prostate gland years ago and now you have cancer in the bone that tests show to be prostate cancer in the bone, you have had a recurrence of prostate cancer. Conversely, if you had prostate cancer years ago and now you have colon cancer, you have developed a new, unrelated cancer, called a "second primary."

How Do Doctors Know Whether a New Cancer Is a Recurrence of a Past Cancer or an Unrelated Second Primary?

Evaluation of a piece of the new cancer under a microscope and with other sophisticated tests tells doctors what kind of cancer it is. In most cases this evaluation can determine whether the new cancer is a recurrence of a prior cancer or an unrelated second primary. When possible, doctors will compare slides of the new cancer with slides of the prior cancer under the microscope to resolve any question about the new cancer's being a recurrence. Occasionally, some uncertainty persists whether a cancer is a recurrence of a prior cancer or a new, second cancer.

Can a Cancer Ever Come Back as a Different Cancer?

Some types of cancer can transform or change into a different form of the same type of cancer when they recur. For example, low-grade lymphoma can go into remission and then recur in a different, high-grade form. Even though the new lymphoma behaves very differently, it is felt to be a recurrence of the original lymphoma and not a second, unrelated primary.

Lymphomas always come back as lymphomas, even if they come back as a different type of lymphoma. Breast cancer recurs only as breast cancer. Prostate cancer recurs as prostate cancer, and so on.

What Is a Local Recurrence?

A local recurrence is recurrent cancer at or near the place of the original cancer. If you had melanoma treated with surgery and you develop a recurrence near your scar, you are said to have a local recurrence.

If I Have a Recurrence in the Future, Can I Ever Be Cured of My Cancer?

Yes. Many people are cured of their cancer after being treated for recurrent cancer.

Recurrence is not a death sentence; it is an illness.

If your original cancer was treatable, there is a good chance that a recurrence will be treatable.

If I Have a Recurrence, Does That Mean That I Was Never Really Rid of My Cancer?

Yes. If you have a recurrence, the assumption is that some cancer cells were not killed by your original treatment and have been hiding for months or years, undetected by all your checkup tests until they multiplied enough to cause you to have detectable cancer.

If I Can Have Undetectable Cancer Cells That Become a Problem Years Later, How Can I Ever Know That I Am Really Free of Cancer?

A big fear of cancer survivors after successful treatment is the fear of recurrence from cancer cells that are not detectable during the period of clinical remission.

It is impossible to guarantee that every last cancer cell is gone. From a realistic, practical point of view, it is only important to know whether you have any cancer cells in your body if

• these cells can cause a problem to you in the future, and
• there is something you can do now to treat these cells or prevent them from developing into significant cancer

Even if you do harbor silent cancer cells, for all practical purposes you are now cancer-free and can remain so for the rest of your life. Our bodies are believed to have an immune surveillance system that can help prevent the development of detectable recurrent cancer by destroying cancer cells that appear in small numbers.

Cancer cells that current technology cannot detect are not affecting your life in any way as long as they remain undetectable. The only danger in this situation is letting your own thoughts or worries about undetected cancer cells affect you in a negative way. It does not help you to worry about the possibility of something you cannot know or do anything about. Survivorship includes accepting the uncertainty of whether any cancer cells are left. See your remission as meaning that you are completely cancer-free unless there is concrete evidence to the contrary.

If you are in remission, and you and your doctors have done everything reasonable to kill any remaining silent cancer cells, you should assume that you are cancer-free and focus on ways to keep yourself healthy.

If Cancer Cells Are So Powerful That They Can Cause Life-Threatening Disease, How Can I Ever Relax Knowing That There Might Be Cancer Cells in Me?

With time and practice, you can learn to lessen worries about leftover cancer cells. Some techniques that will help include

- learning to view cancer cells as the weak, abnormal cells that they are
- learning to regard your body as possessing powerful defenses against cancer cells (this is hard to do soon after cancer treatment: after all, your body allowed the cancer to grow in the first place, and it is weak from treatments)
- focusing on efforts to keep your body healthy and strong
- concentrating on increasing your capacity for acceptance and hope, and decreasing your need for control and perfection

• learning to accept that this is an uncertainty with which you will have to live

We have learned from people who live long lives with certain types of incurable cancer that the threat to their health and life came less from their persistent cancer than from normal age-related changes and illnesses. Even though they had known cancer, their cancer had little effect on their life or longevity unless they let the knowledge of their cancer affect them emotionally in a negative way.

Remind yourself of the patient who was successfully treated for cancer and spent the next forty years physically healthy but worried sick about a possible recurrence. At the age of ninety-eight the patient said, "I guess I really was in remission all these years. I spoiled what could have been forty wonderful years worrying about something that never happened."

Do not lose today by worrying about something you can never know (whether or not you have any leftover cancer cells) or about something that may never happen (recurrence).

PREVENTING RECURRENT AND NEW CANCERS

What Can I Do to Prevent a Recurrence?

There are steps you can take to help prevent recurrence. Specific recommendations for you depend on the type of cancer you had and your medical condition. Areas of potential intervention include

• diet modification
• exercise
• avoidance of exposure to cancer-causing environmental substances
• hormonal therapy

- medicines to prevent recurrence
- aggressive surveillance, such as routine Pap smears, colonoscopies, or mammograms to detect precancerous changes (changes that are not yet cancer but have a high likelihood of becoming cancer)
- removal of precancerous lesions detected by aggressive surveillance

What Is Adjuvant Therapy?

Some types of cancer can be treated with additional therapy after you are in remission, in the hope of "mopping up" any leftover undetectable cancer cells. This additional therapy, called adjuvant therapy, is given with the expectation that it will decrease your chance of recurrence. It is at present available for a number of cancers that are notorious for recurrence.

For example, people with certain types of early breast cancer can be put into remission with surgery and radiation, but are advised to receive adjuvant chemotherapy (a few months of chemotherapy) to kill any cancer cells left anywhere in the body. When adjuvant therapy is an option, it should be considered seriously.

What Is Chemoprophylaxis?

Chemoprophylaxis is the use of medication to prevent a recurrence of cancer, prevent a second cancer that is different from a person's past cancer, or prevent a first cancer in someone who has never had cancer. This is a new and very exciting area of cancer research. Trials are under way to explore medicines believed to offer protection. For example, large-scale studies are in progress to determine whether the use of tamoxifen can help prevent recurrent breast cancer or a new breast cancer in the opposite breast, or whether the use of anti-inflammatory medication can help prevent colon cancer.

There exists no medicine that will prevent all cancers, and it is unlikely that any will ever be found. However, we have every reason to expect to see the development of medicines that will help prevent certain types of cancer, especially in people at a known increased risk.

What Is Supplemental Therapy?

Supplemental therapy is treatment intended to be used in addition to conventional therapy. Examples of supplemental therapies include visual imagery, special diets, vitamins, exercise, counseling, prayer, humor, biofeedback, relaxation, and meditation.

Proponents believe that adding supplemental therapy to your conventional cancer treatments may promote your physical and emotional comfort, enhance your response to conventional therapy, speed your recovery from cancer treatment, and possibly improve your chances against your cancer. The role of supplemental therapy in strengthening the immune system is being evaluated.

Supplemental therapies are never intended to be used as the only therapy when conventional therapy is available. Many people turn to supplemental therapy alone when they have completed conventional therapy and there is no available additional conventional therapy for keeping them in remission. Other people use supplemental therapy alone, with the hope of controlling their cancer, after all conventional therapies have failed.

What Is Visualization?

Visualization is the process of imagining a desired effect or outcome in your mind. Before winding up to throw, baseball pitchers visualize the ball flying through the strike zone. They even visualize throwing strikes while they warm up in the bullpen or relax at home in the evening. Somehow this visualization helps their muscles perform when they are on the mound.

You visualize for healing by imagining your body fixing the body's problem. If you had surgery, you can visualize the incision healing. If you had chemotherapy or radiation, you can visualize the treatment damaging and killing cancer cells, and your white cells killing and clearing away cancer cells.

Your visualization may be fairly realistic if you know what your cancer cells and white cells look like. Visualization is felt to be just as effective if you use simplistic images or even symbols. You may visualize white dots (your white blood cells) gobbling up black dots (your leftover cancer cells or any new cancer cells) the way Pac-Man eats the computer dots.

Visualization can be even more abstract. You may imagine a wave (the cancer treatment and your body's immune system) washing over a beach and then retreating to the ocean, carrying away any debris (cancer cells).

What Is the Role of Visualization in Healing and in Fighting Cancer?

The body is an extremely complex organism. Your mind plays a role in how your body functions. Some research-oriented psychologists and psychiatrists, and a few immunologists and other specialists have speculated that you can affect how well your body fights cancer by visualizing the hoped-for results, just as you can affect how accurately you throw a ball by concentrating on the process. No study to date has shown any significant effect on cure rates or rates of recurrence through visualization. However, visualization in some people does cause measurable improvement in medical problems such as pain, migraine headaches, insomnia, and muscle spasm.

Visualization is a wonderful tool for people in whom it helps alleviate physical and emotional symptoms. As for your cancer, visualization can help decrease negative stress and give you some sense of control.

Visualization can hurt you if you feel guilty when you do not do it or feel responsible if you have medical problems despite genuine efforts to visualize. Visualization is not for everybody.

What Are the Disadvantages of Supplemental Therapy?

Each supplemental therapy has advantages and disadvantages. Even though most supplemental therapies are "nonprescription," they sometimes involve a real risk of significant physical or emotional harm. Discuss with your doctors the medical risks and benefits to you. The pursuit of supplemental therapy requires an investment of your time, energy, or money.

When you believe in the potential benefit of a particular supplemental therapy, you nourish hope and a sense of control. On the other hand, if you feel pressured to pursue supplemental therapy or if you "want" to believe but are actually very skeptical of the benefits, the pursuit may be counterproductive. Under these and other circumstances, various supplemental therapies heighten rather than lessen your anxiety, drain rather than bolster your energy, and cause rather than relieve symptoms.

Make your decisions about supplemental therapy with the same care that you used in choosing your conventional cancer treatments. Find out from knowledgeable people (doctors, nurses, social workers, and counselors) what your options are. Discuss the potential benefits and risks for you, as indicated by reliable data. Information about supplemental therapy will allow you to maximize your resources toward healing.

How Do I Find Out about Supplemental Therapy?

You can learn more about visual imagery, biofeedback, relaxation, and meditation through self-help books and audiotapes or through consultation with a counselor, psychologist, or psychiatrist trained in biofeedback and visualization. A good starting place for self-instruction is Lawrence LeShan's *How to Meditate,* Herbert Benson's *The Relaxation Response,* and Shakti Gawain's *Creative Visualization.*

Information about special diets and vitamins can be obtained from the hospital's nutrition counselor and the American Cancer Society. Dozens of self-help books are available, but the safety and scientific validity of their regimens are extremely variable. If you decide to follow a special diet, be sure to discuss it with your oncologist first.

You can find out about a good exercise program by investigating your local hospital's rehabilitation programs. Although cancer-specific rehabilitation programs are still scarce, you may fit in well with an established heart, lung, or arthritis rehab program, depending on your current physical condition. These same programs may have instructors who can set up an individualized program that you can follow on your own, if you are well enough. Ask your oncologist or internist whether he or she has some guidelines for an exercise program.

There are many forms of counseling and support. Call the local chapter of the American Cancer Society and your hospital's social work department for the names of the various services available in your area. Find out the focus of each of the services and the fee, if any. Some groups function as a forum for the presentation of information, some stress peer support, and others are more psychoanalytically oriented. Individual counseling offers a diversity of approaches, from short-term, crisis-oriented counseling to lengthy, insight-oriented analysis. It is preferable to seek the services of someone well versed in cancer-related issues.

After you find out about the available resources, try a few that sound interesting. Support services and counseling are two areas where you can usually pick and choose. Select the best ones for you.

There are many places to find humor: funny movies, comic and joke books, comedy audiotapes, and stand-up comedy (live and televised). You can borrow "Candid Camera" videos free of charge by writing to Laughter Therapy, Allen Funt Productions, P.O. Box 827, Monterey, CA 93940. Allen Klein's book *The Healing Power of Humor* (1989) teaches you how to use humor to cope with serious problems. Check the yellow pages for any nearby workshops that focus on finding humor in your life.

What Are Clinical Trials?

Studies on new cancer treatments for human volunteers are called clinical trials. The drugs or treatments have already been shown to have anticancer effects in the laboratory. The goal is to find more effective and safer cancer treatments.

Investigational treatments, also called experimental treatments, are not the same as alternative treatments.

Who Runs Clinical Trials?

Clinical trials are overseen by

- the National Cancer Institute (NCI)
- a "cooperative group," an organized group of oncologists from a number of hospitals and clinics who are trained in designing, running, and interpreting clinical trials
- a qualified individual oncologist or group of oncologists in one institution or clinic

Why Would I Want to Enter a Clinical Trial?

A clinical trial can offer you some unique advantages:

- It can provide an opportunity to try newer treatments before they are generally available.
- These new treatments may prove to be your best chance for doing well.
- It can offer a chance to participate in work that helps all cancer survivors, no matter your outcome from the trial or the conclusions drawn from the trial.
- If you are in remission from a cancer with a very high rate of recurrence, and there is no standard therapy to help prevent recurrence, you may want to try to increase your chance of prolonging your remission.

• Some people feel they are watched more closely in a trial, since the investigators have to report on all results.
• Some clinical trials provide all treatment and follow-up at no cost to the patient.

Are People Who Participate in Clinical Trials "Guinea Pigs"?

No. The term has come to be associated with animals or people used against their will for experiments without regard to their safety.

The negative connotations of the term "guinea pig" do not apply to clinical trials. You cannot become a participant in a clinical trial without your written informed consent, let alone without your knowledge. Clinical trials are controlled, informed situations where your short-term and long-term safety are of paramount importance. Except for Phase I cancer experiments, clinical trials offer you the possibility of doing more to treat or prevent cancer than is available with standard therapy.

Many Phase II or III clinical trials offer exposure to cutting-edge treatment and technology before it is routinely available. These treatments are administered by highly trained, highly qualified doctors.

Do Doctors Ever Give Placebos ("Sugar Pills") to Patients?

A placebo is a treatment designed to have no therapeutic effect. You cannot receive a placebo against your will. The only time a doctor prescribes a placebo for a patient is when the patient signs a consent to participate in a trial where some patients are expected to receive placebos.

Some clinical trials are so-called double-blind placebo-controlled studies. In these studies neither the patients nor the doctors know ("double-blind") which patients are getting the new treatment (such as pills or intravenous medicine) and which patients are getting a blank ("placebo," such as a sugar pill or intravenous saltwater). Studies are done this way in order that valid, reliable conclusions may be drawn.

If doctors or patients always knew who was getting the active treatment, they might be inclined to bias their reporting one way or another, even if they were trying to be objective. If treatments were not compared against placebos, you would never know whether an observed advantage was due to the treatment or to some other factor.

Each patient's well-being always takes top priority, even in cases where placebos may be given. Some double-blind placebo-controlled studies are done with patients who are doing poorly and who have no known effective options left. For these patients the only choice is between doing nothing, and dying for sure, and participating in a clinical trial, and perhaps receiving a treatment that may have an effect on their cancer.

Even when patients are in an early-phase trial and the doctors do not expect them to receive any medical benefit from the low doses of the new treatment, the patients who participate in the study enjoy the benefit of feeling that they are contributing to the advancement of cancer care. Investigational therapy allows them to hope that they will respond despite expectations to the contrary. Nourishing hope and giving meaning to the illness are two vital benefits of clinical trials for these people.

Double-blind placebo-controlled trials are also done in patients who are doing well but have nothing available to help decrease the risk of recurrence or other future medical problems. In this situation the people who receive placebos are getting the same treatment (namely, nothing) they would get if they were not participating in the clinical trial.

Why Doesn't Everyone Participate in Clinical Trials?

There are practical reasons why many people do not participate in clinical trials:

- People are unaware of the availability and benefits of trials.
- Trials have limited participation; there may be no space in ongoing trials for a person's particular cancer situation.
- People may not qualify for trials applicable to their type of can-

cer, because of concurrent medical conditions, age, location, or family constraints.

•Certain kinds of clinical trials offer little or no therapeutic benefit.

What Are the Downsides of Clinical Trials?

There are some potential disadvantages to your participating in a clinical trial:

•By definition, not all of the risks and benefits are known ahead of time; there can be unexpected dangers and side effects.

•Doctors have less experience working with new treatments than with standard, established ones.

•You may lose an opportunity for a dependable response from standard therapy if you pursue a clinical trial of therapy that proves to be less successful than standard therapy.

•Clinical trials require an investment in terms of your time, energy, and testing to comply with the required follow-up during and after treatment.

•Hospitalization may be required for some treatments.

•Trials can add to the emotional stress of not knowing exactly which treatment you are getting. As was discussed above, some patients receive a placebo (e.g., an inactive sugar pill) instead of the experimental treatment in placebo-controlled studies. In other studies, you randomly receive either standard treatment or the new treatment. Despite the reassurance that you are receiving treatment that has an anticancer effect, not knowing exactly what treatment you are getting can be stressful.

•Some people feel like "a number" instead of an individual human being.

Although clinical trials increase your potential options, they are not for everyone.

Is It Too Late for Me to Enter a Clinical Trial If I Have Completed a Course of Cancer Therapy and Am Now in Remission?

Studies are being done with treatments that will improve the durability (length of time) of remission. Find out about trials available to you by

- requesting a copy of the latest PDQ (Physician Data Query) related to your type of cancer (this is a service of the National Cancer Institute, available by calling its toll-free number, 1-800-4CANCER)
- asking your oncologist
- calling major cancer centers to inquire about any studies that have not yet been registered with the NCI

What If My Oncologist Discourages Me from Investigating or Participating in a Clinical Trial?

Discuss with your oncologist why he or she opposes your participating in a clinical trial. Consider getting a second opinion from an oncologist who encourages participation in clinical trials but does not participate personally.

It is possible that your oncologist discourages you because he or she is uncomfortable with clinical trials or does not want to "lose you" as a patient to the oncologists running the trial. One would like to hope, rather, that it is because your doctor has your physical and emotional health in mind.

What Is "Informed Consent"?

Informed consent is your written approval to receive treatment *after* you have received information that allows you to understand

- the nature of the treatment
- the purpose of the treatment

• the benefits, short-term and long-term
• the risks, short-term and long-term
• the expense, short-term and long-term

Once I Participate in a Clinical Trial, Am I Obligated to Stay in the Trial?

No. Participation in a clinical trial is totally up to you. You can drop out of the study at any moment without jeopardizing your medical care. You have every right to do what is best for you, physically or emotionally. If, during the study, it becomes obvious that the treatment is not good for you, you will be removed from the study.

However, agreeing to participate in a clinical trial implies a level of commitment. It takes manpower, equipment, and money to run a clinical trial. Information is lost and costs are increased when participants drop out.

What Are Antioxidants?

Antioxidants are micronutrients (substances found in tiny amounts) that serve as the body's primary defense against free radicals and reactive oxygen molecules (two by-products of normal metabolism that are thought to cause damage to normal cells, possibly predisposing the damaged cells to become cancerous). If free radicals trigger the early changes of cancer, then antioxidants would protect patients by mopping up these free radicals.

Antioxidants include

• carotenoids
• beta-carotenes
• vitamin C
• vitamin E

Selenium is an essential component of antioxidant enzymes.

What Are the Facts regarding Antioxidants as Protection against Cancer?

Animal studies suggest a protective role for antioxidants in the fight against various types of cancer, particularly lung and epithelial cancers. We cannot draw conclusions about humans on the basis of animal studies. The results from animal studies help us proceed to human studies in a safe and expeditious manner.

Human studies have shown an association between

- a diet low in carotenoids and an increased risk of lung cancer
- a diet low in vitamin C and an increased risk of oral, esophageal, and stomach cancer
- a diet high in vitamin C and beta-carotene and a decreased risk of cervical dysplasia and oral leukoplakia
- a diet high in vitamin C and a protective effect against cancers of the esophagus, mouth, stomach, pancreas, cervix, rectum, breast, and possibly lung
- low blood levels of beta-carotene and an increased risk of lung cancer
- low blood levels of vitamin C and an increased risk of stomach cancer

These and other data certainly suggest that antioxidants protect against some types of cancer. Well-designed human studies are under way to determine definitively which antioxidants in what dose and form guard against which specific cancers.

What about the Role of Fruits and Vegetables in Protecting against Future Cancer?

Epidemiologic studies have shown that people whose culture is characterized by a diet rich in fruits and vegetables have a lower risk for certain types of cancer than those whose diet is lacking in these foods. In addition, when people who normally eat few fruits and vegetables add fruits and vegetables to their diet, they appear to lower their risk of developing certain cancers. The relationship between eating fruits and vegetables and reducing risk is not just an association; these foods actually do cause changes in the body that protect against cancer.

We do not know whether the benefit is due to the antioxidants in the fruits and vegetables or to some other substances, not present in synthetic supplemental antioxidant pills.

The National Institutes of Health (NIH) is currently conducting many studies in humans to look at the role dietary and supplemental antioxidants play in protecting against future cancers. However, no well-controlled human studies have yet given a definitive answer to the question about the benefit of supplemental antioxidants.

What Should I Do about Antioxidants in My Diet until the Results of Current Studies Are Available?

The current recommendation by the American Cancer Society is to eat four to six helpings of fruits and vegetables daily.

Is There Any Risk to My Taking Supplemental Antioxidants in the Form of Pills, Potions, or Powders, until the Final Word Is Out on the Risks and Benefits?

Yes. Medications, even nonprescription medications, can have serious side effects. Vitamins, especially when taken in high doses (megadoses, many times larger than the U.S. recommended daily allowances), are potentially dangerous.

Since vitamin C is water-soluble, you will excrete any excess in your urine. The risks of taking vitamin C pills include

- stomach irritation
- irritation of the esophagus, especially if the vitamin C is taken just prior to lying down
- oxalate kidney stones in people who are at risk
- interference with certain medications, such as Coumadin

• interference with tests for sugar in the urine and blood in the stool
• miscarriage/fetal deformity

Discuss the use of vitamin C with your oncologist. Specifically, find out whether you have any medical conditions that would affect how much vitamin C you can take safely. There is no general answer to the question "How much vitamin C should I take to prevent any future cancer?" Many people take 1–2 grams (1,000–2,000 milligrams) of vitamin C daily, because they deem this dose safe and effective, but solid recommendations are not yet available.

Vitamin E is a fat-soluble vitamin. Taking more than the U.S. recommended daily allowance of vitamin E can be toxic.

Beta-carotene and carotenoids can impart a yellowish tint to the skin.

Are There Any Vitamins or Other Pills I Can Take to Prevent Cancer?

At this time, there is no pill or vitamin that will prevent cancer in general. You can call the NCI's Cancer Information Service number to see whether any clinical trials are investigating a medicine or therapy that will help prevent the recurrence of your type of cancer or the development of another cancer known to be associated with your type. Your oncologist can keep you informed of these studies, too.

What If I Am Embarrassed to Tell My Doctor about Various Over-the-Counter Preparations I Am Taking to Prevent Cancer?

Many people take over-the-counter to help prevent cancer or treat other conditions. Too often, people neglect to tell their doctors about these medicines, either intentionally or unintentionally. Doctors are aware that many people self-medicate with nonprescription pills and tonics. The more information your doctor has about you, the better the care you will receive. If you tell your doctor about your self-prescribed medications, your doctor

- can take this information into account when evaluating a problem
- can warn you of potential problems or dangers to you
- can advise you about a more effective or safer way to use the over-the-counter medications
- can adjust your prescription medications, if necessary

What Is Alternative Therapy?

Alternative therapy is cancer treatment offered instead of conventional medical therapy, often with the claim that it will give you a better chance against your cancer, with fewer side effects. Alternative therapy is not the same as investigational, or experimental, therapy. Examples of alternative therapy include laetrile (the apricot pit medicine), herbal tonics, homeopathy, acupuncture, and metabolic therapy.

Every conventional therapy's effectiveness against cancer has been determined by numerous rigorous, scientifically sound studies. In contrast, no alternative therapy has been shown in a well-controlled scientific study to be more effective than conventional therapy in curing cancer. All of the well-investigated alternative therapies have been shown to be less effective or ineffective in curing or controlling cancer.

Testimonials documenting the effectiveness of alternative therapies abound. But though exciting and inspiring, they do not constitute scientific evidence. The NIH has established the Office of Alternative Medicine to assess scientifically the value of alternative therapies. The information provided by these studies will enable you to make a rational decision about the role of alternative therapy in your cancer treatment.

People with cancer have been using alternative treatments for thousands of years. Only in the past thirty years have large numbers of people with cancer been cured or enjoyed long survival, and this is due to advances in science and technology. Conventional therapy is far from perfect, but by all rational measures it represents the safest and best treatment for cancer available to you at this time.

Why Would I Consider Alternative Therapy Now, after I Have Completed My Conventional Treatments?

There are many reasons why you may consider alternative therapy:

- You may feel the need to be doing something active to treat your cancer or prevent your cancer from recurring. After completion of conventional treatment, the usual prescription from conventional oncologists is to "wait and see."
- You may feel discouraged with the toll conventional therapy has taken and want to get away from conventional medicine.
- You may feel the need to be followed more closely than conventional therapy recommends, so you see alternative therapy as another setting for closer follow-up.
- After treatment may be the first time you have the energy to look at anything other than the treatment you were getting.
- Well-intentioned friends and family may pressure you to look into alternative therapies.
- A desire for control of your situation may lead you to alternatives.
- You may find the alternative-medicine practitioner more optimistic than your oncologist.
- You may find the setting of alternative medicine more comfortable and soothing than the offices and hospitals of conventional medicine.

What Are the Downsides of Alternative Therapies?

Alternative therapies are not as safe or effective as conventional therapies for the treatment of cancer.

Alternative therapies can hurt you when they are used instead of conventional therapy, because

• you may miss an opportunity to control or cure your cancer
  with effective conventional therapy if you spend critical time
  working with alternative therapy
• you can get a false sense of security that you are being treated
  and followed adequately when in fact you are not
• you may be taking unnecessary risks associated with the therapy
• you may spend a lot of money (there is a long, well-documented
  history of charlatans taking advantage of patients, and it still
  occurs today)

Discuss with your doctor your questions and thoughts about
the role of specific alternative therapies in the treatment of your
cancer.

Is There Any Role for Alternative Therapy in the Treatment of Cancer?

Alternative therapy may offer you another option in the treatment
of some of the problems associated with your cancer and cancer
therapy. For example, some of you may benefit from acupuncture
for relief of pain or other symptoms. The acupuncture is helping
control symptoms and is not affecting the cancer. Discuss your
questions and thoughts about the role of specific alternative therapies for the treatment of specific noncancer problems with your
doctors.

How Do I Know Whether a Treatment Is Quackery?

There are warning signs of possible quackery. The company,
clinic, or people offering treatment

• claim the treatment is harmless, painless,and nontoxic
• use a secret formula that is never revealed and cannot be tested
  or reproduced by anyone else
• explain the treatment's action on the basis of unproven theories
• require patients to follow special diets or intense nutritional

support during and after treatment (the failure of the treatment can then be blamed on the patient's inability to follow the rigorous diet)
- discuss their treatment only in the mass media
- support the success of their treatments with testimonials and anecdotes
- have never done controlled studies to document effectiveness
- are not staffed by certified cancer specialists
- do not require a consent form
- attack the medical establishment

Can I Do Both Conventional and Alternative Therapy Together?

If you learn of an alternative treatment that sounds appealing, get objective information about the risks and benefits. Discuss your findings with your oncologist before you make your final decision about which treatments to pursue.

If you decide to proceed with any alternative therapy, it is best to do so under the auspices of your oncologist, so that your progress can be monitored and you will not offset any benefit of conventional therapy.

If your oncologist adamantly opposes your pursuing simultaneous alternative and conventional medicine, and you feel that you must do both, it is safest for you to find a reputable oncologist who feels comfortable with your proposed treatments.

What Is the Role of the Immune System in Prevention of Recurrence?

Research suggests that an intact immune system plays a role in preventing or delaying recurrence in some types of cancer. Your immune system may do this by detecting and destroying cancer cells before they have a chance to multiply and form a cancer big enough to be measurable.

Simple measures that strengthen your immune system and may help prevent recurrence include

• adequate sleep
• moderate exercise
• good nutrition

Factors that are felt to impair your immune system include

• excessive fatigue
• malnutrition
• major grief
• chronic, unpleasant stress

The popular literature is replete with advice about how to build up your immune system. There is little hard scientific evidence to support the many claims of immune-enhancing measures other than those just reviewed.

Since I Have Had Cancer, Am I at Increased Risk for a Second Cancer (a Cancer That Is Not a Recurrence But a New Cancer)?

For many cancer survivors, the answer is yes. You are at increased risk for a second type of cancer if your cancer treatment is known to cause certain types of cancer. Some courses of radiation therapy and many of the chemotherapeutic agents are associated with an increased risk of leukemia.

You are at increased risk for a second cancer if you had a risk factor for your type of cancer and if this risk factor is also a risk factor for other types of cancer. For example, smoking cigarettes puts you at increased risk of many types of cancer, including cancer of the throat and tongue. If you had cancer of the throat and you used to smoke, you are at increased risk of developing tongue cancer. Be aware that if you continue to smoke after being treated for cancer of the throat, your risk of a second cancer in the head or neck is dramatically higher than it would be if you quit smoking.

You are also at increased risk for a second cancer if your type of cancer is associated with increased risk of other types of cancers. For example, some women who have had breast cancer are at a statistically increased risk of developing ovarian cancer.

How Do I Find Out for Which Cancers I Am at Increased Risk?

You can

- ask your doctor
- call the NCI's Cancer Information Service (1-800-4CANCER)
- call the American Cancer Society

What Can I Do to Prevent Other Kinds of Cancer?

This is an area of intense interest and research. At this time the most important recommendations are to

- avoid sun exposure
- eat cruciferous (cabbage family) vegetables
- avoid obesity
- eat a low-fat diet
- include fiber in your diet
- avoid excessive alcohol
- minimize salt-cured, smoked, and nitrite-cured foods
- eat four to six helpings of fruits and vegetables daily

See also Appendix VII.

What Is the Difference between Something Causing Cancer and Something Being Associated with Cancer?

When something causes cancer, it is directly responsible for changes in normal cells that contribute to their becoming cancerous. For example, exposure to the sun causes skin cells to change in such a way that they can become cancerous.

Something is said to be associated with cancer where there exists a statistical relationship between the event being measured and cancer. This says nothing about whether the associated variable being measured is responsible in any way for the changes in the cell that cause it to become cancerous. For example, there may be an association between playing tennis and skin cancer. Playing tennis does not cause any changes in the body that lead to skin cancer. It is the high sun exposure common to tennis players that is responsible for the increased risk of skin cancer.

What Are Cancer Risk Factors?

Conditions or circumstances that increase your risk—your chance—of getting cancer are called risk factors. The presence or absence of risk factors tells you something about your chance of developing a certain type of cancer; it does not tell you whether or not you will get cancer. Many people with risk factors live to an old age and never develop cancer. Many people with no known risk factors do develop cancer.

Different types of cancer have different risk factors. Examples of risk factors include family history (breast, colon, prostate cancers), heavy alcohol consumption (liver, throat, esophagus, mouth), and cigarette smoking (lung, cervix, mouth).

Why Are Cancer Risk Factors Important?

Risk factors for cancer are important because some can be modified, allowing you to reduce your overall risk. Twin brothers whose father died young of malignant melanoma have the same high risk of sun-induced skin cancer on the basis of their strong family history. One brother works inside and uses sunscreen faithfully whenever he goes outside. He has a lower overall risk of developing malignant melanoma than does his brother, who works as a pool lifeguard and is lax about sun protection. Two smokers who develop tongue cancer have an increased risk of developing throat cancer. The person who quits smoking has a much lower risk of developing a second cancer of the head or neck than does the person who continues to smoke.

Knowledge of your risk factors may affect the way you are screened for certain cancers, thus offering the opportunity for earlier detection and treatment. The presence of risk factors may shift the risk–benefit equation in favor of more frequent screening or the institution of preventive treatment for certain types of cancer.

Are My Relatives at Risk for Developing My Type of Cancer?

Only some cancers run in families. Many cancers do not occur with increased frequency in relatives of people with that type of cancer. Ask your doctor whether your relatives are at any increased risk for certain cancers because of your history of cancer.

Should My Family Members Tell Their Doctors about My Cancer?

It is a good idea for your relatives to notify their doctors of your history, because

- as medical knowledge about family risk changes, your relatives' doctors will already be aware of your history
- your relatives' doctors will be more sensitive to your relatives' concerns about symptoms or tests
- your relatives' doctors can encourage them to follow the cancer prevention recommendations
- your relatives' doctors can modify the recommendations regarding prevention and screening where indicated

If My Cancer Tends to Run in Families, Is There Some Way to Prevent My Relatives from Feeling like Sitting Ducks?

Yes. Although their risk may be increased, even significantly, there is much they can do

- to prevent certain types of cancer
- to detect cancer early
- to have hope in the availability of safe and effective treatment, if they need it
- to live with the uncertainty

Cervical and colon cancer are examples of cancers that are preventable if people at risk have routine screening. Breast cancer, colon cancer, and melanoma are examples of cancers that are very curable if detected and treated early.

Knowledge of family risk can ruin one's quality of life if it causes a sense of hopelessness; knowledge of family risk empowers if it is used to maximize prevention and early detection.

What Is a Gene Probe?

A gene probe is a new and exciting laboratory tool that identifies an abnormality in the genes of the tumor cells or the normal cells. These abnormalities are related to the development of certain types of cancer. In research settings, the gene probe is being used to

- help make specific cancer diagnoses
- help better assess the prognosis

How Will Gene Probes Help Cancer Patients?

When gene probes become available in nonresearch settings, they will have an enormous impact on

- how various cancers are diagnosed and staged
- how the best therapy is chosen for each individual
- what treatment options are available

Knowing which cancers are likely to be cured with relatively little treatment and which are likely to act very aggressively allows the doctors to fit the treatment to the cancer better. Patients whose gene probe predicts that they will do well with little treatment will be spared overtreatment. Patients whose gene probe predicts that the only chance is with very aggressive treatment will perhaps be spared recurrence or a poor outcome from treatment that was not aggressive enough.

Gene probes may allow more sensitive follow-up of cancer, making possible earlier detection of recurrence and, therefore, earlier treatment. Most important, it is hoped that gene probes will provide the path to safe, effective, curative therapy by permitting replacement of defective genes that cause cancer.

How Does the Discovery of a Cancer Gene, Such as the Gene for Colon Cancer, Help Me?

Much fanfare surrounds the announcement of each newly discovered cancer gene, such as the recently isolated gene responsible for hereditary nonpolyposis colon cancer. As has happened after the discovery of other genes, a blood test for detecting this gene is being developed and should be available soon.

Such discoveries help you because they

- can identify which of your relatives carries the gene that puts them at higher risk (relatives with the cancer gene could consider participation in a trial of preventive medicines and measures and could pursue the aggressive screening recommended for those at high risk)
- can identify which of your relatives do not carry the gene, and who are at normal risk for the development of that type of cancer (this will spare many people aggressive screening for and anxiety about a high risk that they do not have)
- offer the hope that a way to correct the defective gene in patients will become available to treat people with cancer, and to prevent this type of cancer from ever developing in those at risk
- contribute to our general understanding of cancer prevention, early detection, and treatment
- define populations with high risk that could, by participating in trials, accelerate the discovery of effective preventive medicines and measures for this type of cancer

What Are the Downsides to the Discovery of Cancer Genes?

A serious danger of these discoveries is that people gain a false sense of security if they are found not to have the gene. Feeling safe, they may forgo measures to prevent and detect early cancer, and they thus risk developing the same type of cancer. No test will become available in the foreseeable future, if ever, that will guarantee freedom from all cancer risk.

If you had, for example, colon cancer, your children could be screened for the gene for hereditary nonpolyposis cancer, which accounts for 15 percent of the cases of colon cancer in America. Even if they are found not to harbor this gene, they are still at risk of developing colon cancer from one of the many other genes (most still undiscovered) that can cause it. Your children can be born without any genes predisposing them to colon cancer, but can develop abnormalities that lead to cancer because of exposure to cancer-causing agents.

The ability to pinpoint people at risk for different types of cancer will inevitably have a great impact on health care economics and politics and transform the insurance industry, whose fundamental principle is shared risk.

These exciting discoveries can lead to disappointment if the hopes for preventive and curative measures for the type of cancer are not fulfilled.

Can These Tests Hurt Me or My Family?

As we saw when the blood tests for Huntington's disease and AIDS became available, the decision whether or not to be tested has complex social, legal, and medical ramifications. You may avoid having the test because you fear

- learning that you carry the gene for a type of cancer for which there are no available measures of prevention
- learning that you carry the gene for a type of cancer for which there are no available measures for early detection
- causing family tensions if some members carry the gene and others do not (which is a likely scenario)
- an altered relationship with family, friends, or co-workers if they are found to have the gene
- difficulty in obtaining or keeping insurance if you are found to carry the gene

- difficulty in obtaining or keeping a job if you are found to carry the gene (the Americans with Disabilities Act does not address gene abnormalities, yet)
- dealing with anything related to your own mortality or imperfections

Professional counselors, doctors, and nurses can help you understand how to use the available tests to your best advantage. From a medical point of view, knowledge is power, no matter how distressing. Your risk is your risk, whether you know what that risk is or not. With a knowledge of your risk, you can take steps to minimize your risk and make better decisions about family, career, and finances. (See the section on statistics, pages 265–66.)

Your risk is not your fate. Knowing your risk allows you to minimize it as much as possible.

What Is Susceptibility Testing?

This is a new branch of genetic counseling that determines a person's susceptibility to cancer, or cancer risk, on the basis of analysis of disease in family members (lineages). As this field becomes more sophisticated, refined tools such as gene probes will be added to the analysis.

What Are the Advantages of Susceptibility Testing?

There are important benefits to susceptibility testing:

- It provides new research data that will lead to a better understanding of cancer and to better treatments.
- It can help identify individuals who should take special precautions or be monitored more aggressively. For example, everyone should be screened routinely for colon cancer. The age at which screening begins, the frequency of screening, and the tests used to screen individuals will depend on their susceptibility to colon cancer. Those with higher susceptibility should be screened more often and more completely.

- It can reassure people who feared being at greater risk for a certain cancer and are found to be at normal risk for that cancer.

What Are the Disadvantages of Susceptibility Testing?

Currently, there are a number of disadvantages to pursuing susceptibility testing:

- It can provide false reassurance that you are not at risk. Someone with a strong family history of breast cancer who is found to be at "normal" risk for breast cancer still has a risk of breast cancer. This person needs to perform self–breast exams and have periodic physician exams and mammograms.
- It can cause great anxiety if you are found to have high susceptibility and if there is nothing you can do to prevent the cancer or pick it up at an early, potentially curable stage.

Your susceptibility is not your fate.

Does Finding Out That I Have a High Susceptibility to a Type of Cancer Help Me Prevent This Type?

With our current level of understanding and preventive treatments, susceptibility testing helps you to increase the chance of detecting a precancerous or cancerous lesion early, but it does not help you make decisions about your lifestyle or your medical care that will prevent cancer. Why? On a practical level, people at low risk will want to employ the available preventive measures (such as diet, weight control, sun avoidance) to decrease their risk further, just as people at high risk will want to decrease their risk with preventive measures.

Studies are under way with treatments whose risk–benefit balance will very likely make them valuable only for patients at high risk. When these treatments become available, susceptibility testing will take on greater practical importance for your efforts to prevent cancer. This will be true for treatments that

- work only if you are at high risk
- are too risky to justify using if you are at normal risk

• are too toxic to justify using if you are at normal risk
• are too expensive to justify using if you are at normal risk

Why Did I Get Cancer in the First Place?

Our bodies are made up of millions of cells that grow, divide, and die in an orderly, controlled manner. This dynamic balance allows us to grow hair and skin, maintain a healthy lining to our digestive tract and airway, respond to physical stresses, and repair injuries.

It is believed that most cancers start out as the loss of control of one single cell. A single cancer cell multiplies and becomes a group of cancer cells whose growth is not controlled by the body's healthy cells, and the balance between cell division and cell death is lost. Over months to years, depending on the type of cancer cell, the cancer grows big enough to be detectable or cause problems.

What causes the first cancer cell to become cancerous is still uncertain. Most likely, a series of events has to occur for that to happen. For example, the cell may be genetically predisposed but will not become cancerous unless it is exposed to certain substances or radiation.

For some cancers that seem to arise in multiple spots at once, there may be many cells that lose control at the same time and give rise to many cancers. These cells "at risk" may be exposed to the final "hit," such as radiation or cancer-causing substance, at the same time, so they all become cancerous at the same time.

Now That I Am Done with Treatment, Do I Need to Look for a Cause for My Cancer?

If you have no obvious risk factors for your type of cancer, discuss with your doctor whether it would be worthwhile to look for something in your environment or diet that may have contributed to your developing your type of cancer—for something like asbestos, which is often associated with cancer of the lung lining. The reasons for this inquiry would be

• to ensure that you are not still exposed to something that is continuing to put you at risk for developing this cancer again

• to make sure others are not being exposed
• to provide data for future research

Nothing will change the fact that you had your cancer. Any effort to look for a cause should be geared toward improving the future for you and others.

2

Aftereffects of Cancer Treatments

"The cancer treatment is worse than the disease." You may think this while or after you struggle with cancer treatments, develop complications following treatments, or suffer permanent problems as a result of them. Is it true?

Despite what you may think, cancer treatment is not worse than the disease. The fundamental fact is that most people with cancer who forgo treatment die from their disease. Without treatment, cancer is not only chronic but also terminal. Cancer treatment has allowed you to avoid a life of pain or debility because of progressive cancer. It has given you a chance for a longer life.

Cancer treatments have progressed dramatically over the past few decades, transforming cancer from a near-certain death sentence to one of the most treatable and curable chronic diseases. Encouraged by the successes, doctors have offered patients increasingly more intensive therapies, such as high-dose chemotherapy and bone marrow transplant. And their strategy has paid off. For the first time there exists a huge population of long-term cancer survivors.

But this undeniable success has been won at some cost. Much to survivors' surprise and disappointment, it is very common to experience ongoing and new symptoms and medical problems after treatments are successfully completed. A small but significant percentage of cancer survivors, though cured of their cancer, live the rest of their lives with permanent medical problems. Another small but significant percentage of long-term survivors develop new medical problems, even new cancers, that are directly related to their prior cancer treatments.

The problem is that many people try to see their cancer as a short-term, temporary disease. When people expect surviving cancer to be like surviving a bout of viral meningitis or a broken leg, they find it hard to deal with longer-term problems related to cancer or its treatment. This view of cancer makes people feel that the cure is worse than the disease. A more realistic view of cancer would help.

Cancer is a chronic disease, like heart disease, arthritis, diabetes, asthma, or kidney stones. For some people, minor changes in lifestyle and regular checkups are all that is required. For them the chronic disease has little impact on daily life, and it is easy to forget about the disease. For others the disease profoundly affects every sphere of daily life. In all cases knowledge helps people improve their quality of life and, possibly, lengthen their lives.

The more you learn about the prevention, recognition, and treatment of medical problems, the more you can do to stay healthy. This holds true for anyone living with chronic disease. Consider the story of two young men in the intensive care unit with their first heart attack. The first man was very cooperative, but as soon as he was well enough, he wanted to leave without hearing any more about his heart problem. He said that he did not want to worry about his heart for the rest of his life. He promised to be faithful with his checkups and stress tests, believing that his doctors would pick up any significant changes. With his diet and smoking habits unchanged, he was at risk for recurrent heart attacks. Moreover, he did not know how to recognize problems. A year later he developed pain-free shortness of breath when he climbed the stairs. He thought he was tired that day or might be coming down with a cold. He did not worry about it, let alone call his doctor. He thought he had to have chest pain if he had a heart problem. That night he suffered a massive heart attack.

The other man made every effort to learn about his heart disease. He made changes in his diet, exercise program, work schedule, and over-the-counter medications to minimize his risk of future heart problems. A year later, when he developed some indigestion after mowing the lawn, he went straight to the emergency room. Even though he had no chest pain, he knew that his symptoms could be a warning sign of an impending heart attack. His knowledge saved his life.

You may prefer to stay ignorant of the potential short- and long-term aftereffects of your cancer treatment, because learning about problems makes you feel anxious, angry, or depressed. Anyway, you think to yourself, most cancer survivors do not have long-term medical problems. If only one in a thousand develops a certain complication, why should I learn about it and worry about it, if it is not likely to happen?

The reason to learn about aftereffects of your cancer treatment is that a problem *could* arise. Learning about your cancer is a little like buying fire or theft insurance. You do not want to collect, and you hope never to collect. Most people do not collect. You buy the policy because you *could* need it someday. While you are choosing it, thinking about the possibility of needing it may cause anxiety. Once you have purchased it, you forget about it. After a while, when someone else has a fire or a theft, you will feel reassured that you are covered.

There is a difference between knowing about aftereffects and becoming fixated on them. You may feel quite anxious, worried, or upset while you learn. Once you absorb the information, you can put it away until you need it, if ever. You have to accept a level of anxiety during the hours that you learn about aftereffects in exchange for years of comfort provided by knowing that you are prepared to prevent problems and to recognize them when they are most curable.

If you are someone who prefers to deal with life's challenges by stamping out fires as they flare up, or if you find thinking about potential problems unbearable, this chapter may not be for you. If you think that you would like the information but cannot handle it right now, because you are too tired, fearful, emotional, or just feeling particularly vulnerable, save this chapter for later. Let someone read it for you. When you feel ready, read it yourself.

Learning about recovery from treatment and potential future problems can turn your fear into something useful. You will be more prepared for common symptoms and problems that arise. You can take steps to help prevent or minimize certain problems. You will understand what is happening and be able to participate in your evaluation and treatment. Most important, you will avoid suffering from treatable problems that were neglected because of misinformation or lack of information.

Knowing what to expect after you complete your treatments will allay some of your anxiety. You will be less worried about fatigue, joint pain, or diarrhea, if you know that these symptoms are expected and temporary for someone in your medical situation. Knowledge will help you recognize problems early and know when to get help. A man was treated successfully for lung cancer. Months later he developed a cough. He had never been sick before his cancer, and he explained his refusal to have the cough evaluated by saying, "I am in remission." When, months later, he saw his doctor, he found out that he had a common complication from his radiation that resolved quickly with medication. The cough, and everyone's worry about the cough, was unnecessarily prolonged. A lot of precious energy was wasted in coughing, trying not to worry about it, and dealing with the family stress it caused.

Use this chapter as a form of health insurance. Let the information relieve some of your anxiety by helping to resolve confusion or uncertainty about your symptoms or medical problems. Remember, do not try to diagnose or treat your own medical problems. Use this information to help you recognize problems and work as a partner with your doctors and nurses.

What Are "Late Effects" or "Aftereffects" of Cancer Treatment?

"Late effects" and "aftereffects" are terms used interchangeably to describe any changes or problems that occur after completion of cancer treatment and are due to your cancer or to the treatment you received. These changes and problems can occur weeks, months, or many years after completion of cancer treatment. Technically, there are four different types of aftereffects:

- *Delayed effects* are expected changes that are measurable weeks to months after cancer treatment. Examples of delayed effects include persistent anemia, fatigue, and anxiety following chemotherapy.
- *Delayed complications* are problems that occur only sometimes and appear weeks to months after cancer treatment. Examples of delayed complications include radiation pneumonitis (lung inflammation from radiation), infection related to persistent low blood counts following chemotherapy, and a severe anxiety disorder following any cancer treatment.
- *Late effects* are expected changes that are measurable months to years after cancer treatment. Examples include skin changes following radiation that allow easy sunburn and early menopause following chemotherapy.
- *Late complications* are problems that occur only sometimes, and first appear months to years following cancer treatment. Examples include bowel obstruction from radiation-induced scarring in the abdomen and the development of a second cancer following bone marrow transplantation.

Be sure what definitions are being used when you read or hear about posttreatment problems.

Compared with what we know about the immediate medical effects of cancer treatment, we have relatively little information on its late effects. This is because long-term survivorship is a relatively new phenomenon. However, interest in the field is growing fast. Many studies are under way that promise to provide valuable information about the prevention, diagnosis, and treatment of late effects.

What Causes the Aftereffects of Chemotherapy?

Many of the symptoms or problems you may experience in the first one to two years after completion of chemotherapy are directly due to your chemotherapy. For instance, strong drugs designed to control cancer cells, i.e., chemotherapy, can cause various changes in your blood, such as anemia, which makes you feel weak and tired, or low white blood cell counts, which put you at increased risk for certain infections. Some chemotherapy treatments can affect hormone-producing organs such as the ovaries and testicles. Hormone changes can produce a variety of different side effects, including changes in your emotions and sense of well-being. Some chemotherapy can cause temporary or permanent damage to other organs, such as liver inflammation or weakened kidneys. This damage can affect your stamina or appetite, your capacity to handle medications, and your risk of certain infection.

Other symptoms and problems following chemotherapy are related only indirectly to the treatments. For example, chemotherapy-induced changes in taste sensation may cause you to eat less. This, in turn, can result in vitamin deficiencies and malnutrition. Fatigue, a common aftereffect of chemotherapy, can be due in part to the cumulative effects of the demands of healing (all the places that had cancer are now healing and either returning to their pre-cancerous state or developing a cancer-free scar).

Some of your symptoms are caused, or worsened, by the experience of having had cancer and chemotherapy, and are not really due to the chemotherapy itself. For example, the emotional stress and change in your sleep patterns can cause fatigue and irritability.

How Does Chemotherapy Cause Late Effects (Changes Seen Months to Years after Completion of Chemotherapy)?

Chemotherapy causes many changes in your body. Some of them are detectable during the months when you are receiving your chemotherapy. Others are first detectable weeks, months, or even years after you received your last dose of chemotherapy. Normal age-related changes, infections, or the development of other medical problems, such as diabetes, may make a chemotherapy-related change more obvious. For example, if you suffer subtle hearing loss as a result of your chemotherapy, you may not notice it until years later, when the effect of age-related hearing loss is added on.

Changes caused by chemotherapy that can result in aftereffects include

- changes in normal cells that cause them to become cancer cells; for example, causing leukemia or solid tumors
- changes in the reproductive organs (e.g., ovaries, testicles); for example, causing sterility and menopause
- changes in other hormone-secreting organs (e.g., adrenal glands)
- changes in the heart muscle; for example, caused by high-dose Adriamycin
- scarring of the lung; for example, caused by bleomycin, mito-mycin-C, BCNU (Carmustine), or cyclophosphamide
- injury to kidneys; for example, caused by cisplatin
- injury to nerves; for example, caused by vincristine or cisplatin
- changes in the brain; for example, caused by methotrexate, when given into the spinal fluid

Does Everyone Who Received Chemotherapy Develop Late Effects?

No. Just as everyone's experience with chemotherapy is different, everyone's experience with late effects is different. No two bodies react in exactly the same way. Moreover, two people can have a similar late effect but experience it very differently. For example, most people would tolerate a subtle loss of sensation in their fingertips without much difficulty. However, the same change in a blind person or a violinist could be devastating.

What Factors Influence Whether Chemotherapy Causes Aftereffects?

Many factors influence what aftereffects you may experience following chemotherapy. They include

- the kinds of medicines administered
- the total dose of each medicine received

- the route of therapy, such as by mouth, into a vein, or into the spinal fluid
- the duration of therapy
- the other therapies your body has been exposed to before, during, or after your chemotherapy (e.g., radiation)
- the condition of your kidneys, heart, lungs, or skin before your treatment
- the presence of other medical problems before, during, or after your treatments, such as diabetes, asthma, or hypertension
- your nutritional status
- the administration of other medications
- the presence of infection
- your age at the time of chemotherapy
- your body's ability to heal after exposure to the chemotherapy
- your level of physical fitness before, during, and after chemotherapy

What Causes the Aftereffects of Radiation Therapy?

Many factors contribute to the aftereffects often seen in the first year or so after radiation. Radiation causes damage to rapidly dividing tissue in the parts of the body exposed to the radiation, such as the lining of the digestive tract, the lining of the airway, and the skin. This is seen as a dry mouth, a sore throat, trouble in swallowing, a cough, and a radiation "sunburn."

Radiation causes generalized changes in the blood and immune system. This can be seen as anemia (low red blood cell counts) and low white blood cell counts.

Changes that are not due directly to the radiation but that commonly occur during and after radiation treatments include

- changes in nutritional status and eating habits
- changes in activity level (deconditioning)
- changes in sleep patterns
- an increase in emotional stress
- pain or discomfort

•energy demands of healing (every place that had cancer is now healing to return to its precancerous state or become a scar)

How Does Radiation Cause Late Effects (Changes Seen Months to Years following Completion of Radiation)?

Late effects of radiation are due to changes in the radiated regions of your body that occur during and after your radiation. Some of the changes that can result in late effects include

•changes in the circulation that cause malfunctioning, scarring, or narrowing of an organ
•loss of normal cells from an organ
•changes in normal cells that cause them to become cancerous, especially the bone marrow (leukemia) and soft tissue (sarcoma)
•changes in the thyroid that predispose to hypothyroidism (too low thyroid) or hyperthyroidism (too high thyroid)
•scarring of the lungs
•changes in the small vessels of the brain causing cognitive deficits (thinking problems)
•damage to the bone marrow that causes low blood counts

Except for the short-term changes in the blood counts and immune system, radiation causes changes and problems only in the areas that were radiated. You will not develop radiation-induced thyroid problems if your thyroid gland was not radiated.

Is There Any Interaction between the Late Effects of Chemotherapy and Radiation Therapy?

Sometimes. There are potential interactions for various combinations of chemotherapy and radiation when given together or sequentially. Some chemotherapeutic agents will cause a flare-up reaction of the area radiated weeks, months, or years prior to the chemotherapy. For example, a region of the skin, lung, kidney, or brain that was radiated can become inflamed following the administration of certain chemotherapy.

What Causes the Physical Aftereffects of Surgery?

Most aftereffects of surgery are experienced immediately and resolve within weeks. Aftereffects are due to

- the anesthesia
- the energy demands of healing of the surgical incision (inside and outside)
- changes in eating habits (e.g., not eating before surgery, eating less after surgery)
- changes in activity level
- pain
- a change in sleep patterns
- the need for new medications or changes in medications, especially pain medications
- the adjustment to an amputated or damaged body part, such as a surgically altered lung, breast, kidney, or segment of intestine or stomach
- emotional stress
- hormonal changes caused by lost organ function, such as the infertility, metabolic changes, and psychological changes that follow castration, or the metabolic imbalance following removal of parathyroid glands

Does How I Fared with My Cancer Treatment Give Any Clues Whether or Not I Will Have Serious Late Effects?

No. Severe problems during your cancer therapy, such as mouth problems, extreme low blood counts, or pneumonia, can be followed by no late effects. An absence of problems during treatment can be followed by significant late effects.

If Cancer Treatment Causes Complications and Late Effects, Why Don't Doctors Give Lower Doses of Treatment?

All cancer treatment seeks to strike the best balance between the cure or control of the original cancer and the prevention of complications from the therapy.

If too little cancer therapy is administered in the hope of sparing patients late effects, too many people will die from treatable or curable cancer because of undertreatment. Giving high-dose cancer therapy to everyone in the hope of avoiding undertreatment for the original cancer runs the risk that too many people will die from their treatment or survive with an unacceptably compromised quality of life.

Finding the optimal treatment for each individual patient is like walking a tightrope. Too little cancer treatment for the individual may mean dealing with persistent or recurrent cancer. Too much treatment may mean dealing with debilitating or life-threatening complications. Finding the right amount of treatment to maximize control or cure of your cancer and minimize treatment-related risks is a delicate balancing act.

Was My Treatment Worse Than My Original Disease?

No. If left untreated, most cancers will grow and cause symptoms such as pain, nausea, shortness of breath, and weakness. Uncontrolled cancer causes problems, such as bleeding, respiratory distress, bowel obstruction, infection, and malnutrition, that lead to death. No matter how difficult your cancer treatment, and no matter how many short- and long-term aftereffects you suffer from your treatment, your original cancer, if left untreated, would have become worse than your treatment.

You were treated aggressively to prevent your cancer from becoming a threat to your health and life. If you were diagnosed before you had any significant symptoms or problems, your treatment may have been worse than your early cancer. But it was not worse than the problems your cancer would have caused if it had not been arrested. Compare your treatment-related problems with those that would have developed with untreated cancer.

Why Did I Receive a Treatment That Has Known Late Effects?

Your cancer was a clear and present danger to your health and life. The treatment you received was felt to offer you the best chance of life, with an acceptable risk of future problems, given the treatment options available at the time you were diagnosed.

Your cancer treatments were given to you to protect you from the health- and life-threatening effects of untreated cancer.

Cancer treatments are improving daily. When you see better and safer treatments become available, remind yourself that they

- were not options for you at the time you were treated
- will be available for you if you ever need them in the future
- can be used to treat other people with your type of cancer

Your treatment decisions were based on the best information about the available choices. You did your best.

Do All People Develop Late Effects or Late Problems from Their Cancer Treatment?

No. Although you may have an increased risk for developing certain problems, most cancer survivors do not develop these problems. For example, if the normal risk for developing a certain medical problem is 1 in 5,000 and your cancer treatment puts you at ten times the usual risk, your risk becomes 10 in 5,000. Statistically speaking, this is a much higher risk than if you did not have your cancer treatments, but the absolute risk is still very small.

Are Late Effects Preventable?

As more is learned about late effects, efforts can be made to prevent them by

- adjusting the treatment to be as effective as possible in curing the original cancer while minimizing the chances of creating late effects. Advances in the techniques of radiation therapy allow a more effective killing of cancer cells with less damage to surrounding normal tissue.
- taking measures to protect against late effects. Smoking causes changes in blood vessels that worsen the changes from radiation. Stopping smoking reduces the damage to normal tissue from radiation.
- investigating potential medicines and treatments that do not interfere with killing the cancer cells but help protect the normal cells against the damaging effects of cancer therapy. Several such studies are currently in progress.
- exploring and perfecting medicines or therapies that can be administered after the completion of therapy and that can stabilize exposed normal cells, making them less likely to turn cancerous themselves.
- taking measures to minimize added injury or risk to tissue injured by cancer therapy. Skin that has been radiated is especially vulnerable to the damaging effects of exposure to the sun.
- being alert to situations that trigger late effects. After the patient has received bleomycin or mitomycin-C (two types of chemotherapy), high-dose oxygen can trigger lung injury and thus should be used only when absolutely necessary.

You do not need to become an expert on all of the medical effects of all of your treatments. The way for you to minimize your chances of developing late effects is to

- know the names and amounts of all your treatments
- remind the doctors, anesthesiologists, and dentists who treat you of all treatments you received. Remind them before every treatment; do not assume that they remember prior discussions.

FATIGUE

What Is Fatigue?

Fatigue is defined as a feeling of weariness during or following exertion. It is a common symptom after completion of cancer treatments and can be experienced as any combination of

- feeling tired
- lack of energy or stamina
- difficulty in staying awake
- inadequate physical or emotional energy to respond to signals or problems
- difficulty in concentrating or in learning new information
- poor memory
- excessive yawning
- irritability or emotional lability (ever-changing emotions, such as crying spells or bursts of anger)
- loss of interest in people and things around you
- decreased sexual desire

Fatigue can be subtle or debilitating, constant or fluctuating. It can appear by itself or in association with other symptoms such as headache.

What Causes Fatigue?

Fatigue is a frightening symptom for survivors because they know that cancer can cause fatigue. However, many changes and problems *other than cancer* cause fatigue after recovery from treatment. The most common causes are

- medications such as those used to treat nausea, pain, insomnia, anxiety, depression, high blood pressure, or seizures
- anemia
- chemical imbalances such as a low blood level of potassium caused by prior cancer or treatment

- hormonal changes such as those of menopause, low thyroid, or diabetes
- the physical drain from your body's efforts to heal tissue damaged by the treatments and to clear dead and dying cells
- the effect of substances released by the cells killed or damaged by your treatments
- circulation or heart problems that interfere with the supply of oxygen and energy materials to your organs
- respiratory (breathing) difficulties that interfere with the supply of oxygen to your organs
- physiological changes in your nervous system caused by your prior cancer or treatment
- underlying disease unrelated to your cancer (heart, lung, kidney, musculoskeletal, liver, neurological, or other disease)
- infection in which toxic products are generated or your metabolism is altered, such as by a fever
- emotional factors such as anxiety, depression, frustration, boredom, or conflict
- malnutrition (deficiency of carbohydrates, proteins, minerals, or vitamins) caused by energy requirements of your body that exceed the supply of energy
- interferons or other biological response modifiers that are sometimes given to help maintain a remission (treatment that continues for months, years, or indefinitely after remission is achieved)
- changed sleep patterns
- deconditioning due to inadequate exercise
- overexertion that results in an accumulation of metabolic waste products such as lactic acid
- intake of alcohol, caffeine, or nicotine
- postcancer fatigue (see the next section)

After you complete radiation therapy or chemotherapy, your blood tests, X rays, and scans may all return to normal and yet your fatigue may persist. Under these circumstances, you may have postcancer fatigue (see the next section), which is real, expected, and usually temporary.

You may experience steady tiredness from month to month, as some problems diminish or resolve, others worsen, or new ones develop. In other words, the degree of tiredness may remain the same even though its causes have changed. Anemia may resolve (lessening fatigue) as lung function worsens (exacerbating it). And since malaise also can be the symptom of recurrent cancer or other serious problems, it is critical that you keep your doctor informed. Otherwise you may miss the opportunity for the early diagnosis of recurrent cancer, infection, weakened kidneys, heart failure, or other treatable problems.

In addition, you and your disease can remain unchanged, but your fatigue pattern may change, for unexplained reasons.

Can My Fatigue Be Related to Decreased Sexual Function?

Fatigue is intimately related to sexual function and desire. Many of the problems that cause fatigue, such as low estrogen or testosterone levels, also impair libido and sexual function. Keep your doctor aware of any change in sexual function, because it will help him or her determine the cause and appropriate treatment for your fatigue as well as your diminished sexual function and desire.

Grief, so common during recovery, is a physiological as well as psychological process that can cause both decreased libido and listlessness. As you grieve your losses, you may have no interest in sex for a while. However, if this lack of interest persists, consult with your doctor because physical or emotional issues other than grief may be responsible for it.

On a practical level, if your daily activities sap every last ounce of your energy, none is left for sex. In addition, the ongoing stress of dealing with the limitations imposed by your low energy can lead to chemical or hormonal changes in your body that manifest themselves as diminished sexual function. These changes can occur despite a positive attitude, emotional stability, and optimal social circumstances.

However, as will be discussed below (pages 148–56), human sexuality is a highly complex phenomenon. Since sexual interest and function are influenced by your environment and emotional state, fatigue may indirectly inhibit them. For example, relationships strained by your lack of enough energy to perform (housework, child care, or job) are less conducive to sexual enjoyment.

Anxiety, low self-esteem, and fear about your changed body sometimes, *subconsciously,* may lead you to avoid sexual activity through crippling fatigue. Recognizing when this is a contributing factor will help you deal with the real issue: adjusting to your changed body image. Resolution of this problem will encourage a return to normal sexual activity.

While you were being treated for cancer, significant limitations may have prevented sexual activity. Hospitalization, severe pain, intractable nausea, and treatment-induced lethargy prevent sexual relations no matter how strong the desire. These limitations, lifted during remission, can leave their mark: you and your partner are less spontaneous and comfortable in relating sexually. Prolonged abstinence or near-abstinence may cause you to get out of the habit.

If during your treatment phase you had pain that was exacerbated by sexual activity, initiating sex or even thinking about it may trigger a conditioned type of anxiety or inability to function, even though the pain is now gone completely. This complaint usually responds to appropriate treatment. It is similar to a woman's meeting her chemotherapy nurse in a grocery store ten years after the end of treatment and immediately getting nauseated and throwing up. (Needless to say, the encounter doesn't make the nurse feel very good, either.)

Fatigue and diminished sexual function are often interrelated. Attention to both will facilitate their improvement.

What Should I Do If Fatigue Is Interfering with My Sexual Function?

Explore the various causes of diminished sexual function, and address those that apply to you. You cannot force sexual function to return quickly, but you can facilitate its return by

- seeing the change as one of the many aftereffects of your cancer experience
- aiming to develop a sexual balance with your partner that may, of necessity, be different from the earlier balance
- accepting the reality that things will be different for a while, if not forever
- trying to be patient
- developing new ways to express affection and sexuality that do not deplete your energy reserves

Remember that your partner, too, has to adjust to the changes brought on by your illness and recovery. He or she may be dealing with many of the factors that are bothering you, such as grief, anxiety, depression, anger, and depleted emotional and physical reserves. Moreover, a solution or balance that works for you may be unacceptable to your partner. Simple caressing may satisfy your needs, but not your partner's. Anytime that two people's needs and goals get out of synchrony, honest and caring dialogue helps them approach a mutually acceptable solution.

Before blaming any sexual difficulties on fatigue or the cancer experience, reflect on how things were going prior to your illness. Current difficulties may merely be the continuation or reappearance of old problems. If you had sexual difficulties before, chances are that the stress of your treatment and recovery has not helped (although some people *do* settle problems and attain a new level of intimacy during the cancer treatment phase). Apply the insights and tools gained during your treatment and recovery to any current difficulties; long-standing problems may, at last, be resolved.

Sexuality can be difficult to discuss with your partner under the best of circumstances. Encourage a sharing of feelings and concerns. If you cannot figure out how to broach the subject with your loved one, or if you have tried unsuccessfully, ask your doctor or nurse for referral to someone skilled in dealing with the effects of illness on relationships. Time alone is often a great healer. But why wait? Quality counseling may enable you and your partner to reach a new equilibrium faster. This not only prevents or minimizes the added stress of sexual difficulties; it also gives you the benefit of the psychological lift and emotional comfort of resumed relations.

When Will My Energy Return to Normal?

How quickly your energy level returns to normal will depend on

- your energy level before you were diagnosed
- the type of cancer treatment you received
- the intensity of cancer treatment
- the duration of cancer treatment
- the type, intensity, and duration of any pain
- the presence of any depression, anxiety, or other emotional distress
- the soundness of your nutrition
- the quality of your sleep
- your hormonal balance
- ongoing medical problems, such as infection or wound healing, kidney failure, or heart failure
- your ability to pace yourself
- your level of fitness
- factors that we cannot measure (cellular changes, your will to live, and so on)

In general, people need two days to two weeks to recuperate from uneventful minor surgery. Allow two weeks to three months for recovery from uneventful major surgery. Radiation therapy can cause fatigue lasting for one to five months after the completion of therapy, depending on the area that was exposed and the total amount of radiation received. Chemotherapy lasting four or more months is usually associated with fatigue that persists for six months to a year or two after the last treatment, depending upon the agents used, the intensity of treatment, and the duration of treatment. As progress has been made in the safe administration of aggressive chemotherapeutic regimens for previously uncontrollable cancers, fatigue has become a more common, and often more debilitating, problem.

In general, the more intense your treatment, the worse your symptoms. Exposure to more than one type of treatment—such as surgery plus radiation, or radiation plus chemotherapy—has a cumulative effect on energy levels. The presence of other fatigue-inducing factors, such as anemia or malnutrition, will exacerbate that due to cancer treatments.

These guidelines are very general. Many patients, usually those requiring relatively little treatment, bounce back to their precancer state of well-being quickly. Most people who have received a significant amount of radiation or chemotherapy take weeks to months to feel well consistently. Fatigue is universal after rigorous treatments such as high-dose radiation or chemotherapy requiring a bone marrow transplant, and it usually persists for at least a year or more.

Recognize that many unmeasurable factors affect energy, making it impossible to provide an accurate prediction of when you will feel normal in terms of energy. Although for most survivors fatigue is a temporary, if protracted, problem, for some it becomes a chronic disability, especially if factors that contribute to it persist indefinitely.

Two thirty-six-year-old women had the same type of leukemia and were simultaneously given the same treatment regimen prior to their bone marrow transplants. One year later they were both in remission, but one felt well; her bone marrow had recovered completely, and her blood counts were normal. The other suffered from debilitating exhaustion because her bone marrow had never recovered fully, and she remained anemic. Unless her bone marrow recovered—an increasingly unlikely event the longer she went without improvement—low energy levels would continue to be an issue.

Your treatment changed your body's physiology, at least temporarily. Something else changed during your treatment, something that had nothing to do with cancer or treatment: you got older. The same intense treatment regimens that are administered over many months, or even years, demand a longer time interval between "before" and "after." The passage of six to eighteen months of treatment plus another six to twelve months of recovery means you will be comparing yourself to how you were at least one to two years earlier. If you felt poorly before your diagnosis, the time since you last felt well is even longer. A few years might not seem like a lot of aging, but healthy twenty-year-olds often notice a difference in stamina compared with when they were eighteen; forty-year-olds, compared with when they were thirty-eight; or sixty-five-year olds, compared with when they were sixty-three.

What If I Am Regaining My Energy More Slowly Than Others Who Were Treated at the Same Time?

Your specific circumstances before, during, and after treatment, as well as your reaction (physical and emotional) to your circumstances are unique, thus making your recovery pattern unique. No one can tell you how you feel or should feel. However you feel is how you feel. Comparing your energy level with that of a survivor who is enjoying a faster or smoother recovery, or with yours before your illness, does not help you (unless it provides hope and inspiration). The issue is how to get you feeling as well as possible now and in the future. Work toward developing a new sense of well-being and good health, as opposed to trying to get back to where you were before cancer. Focus on ways you can improve your energy.

When My Energy Comes Back, Will It Return Suddenly?

Like most everything else about recovery from cancer treatment, the manner in which your energy returns will be very individual. For most people, improvement is gradual. You will begin to have days with more energy, often followed by days with less energy. In general, the trend is toward more and more energy, provided there are no setbacks, such as minor illness, surgery, injury, or emotional stress. Occasionally people report a sudden return to their usual level of energy.

Is There Anything I Can Do to Help My Energy Come Back Faster?

Many measures will help you feel better while your doctors are evaluating and treating the various problems that may be contributing to your fatigue. They may not be high-tech, like chemotherapy or surgery, but they work. Try to

- get adequate rest (when you feel fatigued)
- eat well-balanced meals and snacks, as advised by your doctor or a nutritionist to meet your posttreatment nutritional demands (your protein, fluid, and calorie requirements remain elevated for a while after treatment is completed in order that your body can repair tissue damaged by the treatments and clear the waste from the dead cancer cells)
- avoid excessive physical and emotional stress
- prioritize your activities so that you can maintain an energy-conserving schedule (you may need help to do this)
- continue to delegate tasks to others so that you can continue to conserve your energy for healing
- continue to obtain help, as needed, in such activities as making meals, carpooling, taking out the garbage, and bathing
- begin a doctor-approved exercise program
- address your feelings of anxiety, fear, depression, grief, and anger
- discuss the role of antidepressants in the treatment of your fatigue
- discuss vitamin and nutritional supplementation with your doctor

What Should I Tell My Doctors about My Fatigue?

It is important that you keep your doctors informed about your energy level. Describe in concrete terms how tired you are: "When I sit down to dinner, I'm too exhausted to lift the fork to my mouth," "After I get my kids ready for school, I have to lie down," or "I'm fine when I get to work, but by eleven I can't concentrate and need to close my eyes."

Describe the pattern of your fatigue: how often it occurs, when it occurs, how severe it is, what triggers or aggravates it, what prevents or alleviates it, and what the overall trend is (e.g., getting worse or better the past few weeks, the same as it has been since treatment ended). Is it worse in the morning or the afternoon? When you are hungry or full? When you do or do not get exercise? On workdays or schooldays or weekends?

Explain to your doctor how your energy limitations are affecting you on a practical level. A single mother of two young children may be unable to take care of them because of her fatigue, or she may be unable to get the rest she needs to offset the fatigue. In contrast, a widowed grandmother may be able to satisfy her physical and emotional needs by adjusting her daily schedule to accommodate her slowed pace and increased need for sleep.

Your doctor also needs to know how you are being affected emotionally. Do you fear that the fatigue indicates persistent or recurrent cancer? Is your inability to do what you want or need to do making you feel depressed? Is it causing problems at work or home?

Can Anything Be Done to Alleviate My Fatigue If My Doctors Find Nothing Wrong and I Am Following All the Measures Described Above?

With the growth of the population of long-term survivors and with the progress in the prevention and treatment of other problems seen after cancer, such as nausea and malnutrition, the issue of fatigue has moved into the spotlight. Research into its causes, prevention, and treatment is under way. Until answers are found, you must direct your attention to

- correcting all treatable causes (such as anemia, malnutrition, or depression)
- taking steps to prevent problems that cause it
- having your doctors adjust your medications, whenever possible

• developing a healthy daily routine that includes adequate rest
• adjusting to your limitations

Support services can help you adapt and adjust to your fatigue so as to maximize your overall recovery. Loss of energy, like loss of a limb, must be grieved. Adjustments must be made. All of this takes time, energy, and patience.

What Can I Do If My Fatigue Seems out of Proportion to the Treatment I Received or Seems to Be Lasting Too Long?

When fatigue persists, it is common to worry, consciously or unconsciously, that you have cancer again. Remind yourself that many problems other than cancer cause fatigue. In most cases where tests indicate that you are in remission, there is a good explanation other than cancer. Sometimes, however, the fatigue seen in disease-free cancer survivors has no explanation.

Keep your doctor and nurse aware of how you feel, even if your tiredness was addressed before and all treatable causes were ruled out. Although you may feel exactly the same, the explanation may have changed.

One man who was in remission after completing a course of radiation complained of lassitude, feeling cold, getting winded easily, and poor concentration and memory. A complete workup indicated that his thyroid was definitely normal, but he was mildly malnourished. His doctors reassured him that he was experiencing a common aftereffect of radiation in addition to the effects of malnutrition. As the weeks went by, he stuck to a prescribed diet and regained his weight; yet he continued to feel the same. After four months without any improvement, his doctor rechecked his thyroid blood tests; lo and behold, they were low. He had developed hypothyroidism (low thyroid) after the first evaluation, and his symptoms resolved after he took a thyroid medicine for a few weeks. Although he felt the same immediately after completion of his radiation as four months later, the cause of his fatigue was different each time.

Another patient suffered debilitating fatigue following her bone marrow transplant. A complete evaluation showed that she was adjusting well to her situation and was not depressed. Her fatigue was attributed to mild anemia and the physical aftereffects of intensive chemotherapy and radiation therapy. She followed all the advice given to her about diet, exercise, and rest. Over the next year her fatigue became less debilitating but was disturbingly persistent. A reevaluation determined that she had developed significant depression, which was manifesting itself chiefly as fatigue, a not uncommon occurrence after bone marrow transplantation. She responded dramatically to medication and counseling and is now doing beautifully without any medication.

Have your doctor or nurse advise you on specific ways to improve your diet, sleep patterns, exercise schedule, work level, and stress level. Support groups and counselors (social workers, psychologists, etc.) can offer invaluable advice and support in these areas.

If I Have Trouble Tolerating Fatigue, Why Is This?

Feeling drained all the time can impair your quality of life in a major way. After having tolerated other, more dramatic symptoms or problems, you might expect fatigue to be a minor nuisance. However, it is challenging because of its effect on all aspects of your life. Lack of energy and all its repercussions represent ongoing loss.

After cancer the rhythm of routine and the feeling of satisfaction that comes from completing tasks helps you feel that your life is getting back to normal. Unfortunately, you may neglect some tasks, or do them poorly, if you are straining just to fulfill daily responsibilities. A sense of routine may seem elusive if you lack adequate emotional or physical reserves to deal with everyday interruptions and problems (such as spilled milk, misunderstandings with friends, or news of a friend's heart attack). Without the satisfaction of completing tasks or the comfort of a routine you may experience a lingering sense of being sick and out of control.

The stress of knowing that you cannot do as much as before

is augmented by the stress caused by the consequences of this incapacity. For example, added to the inconvenience of your child's not having clean clothes because you were too exhausted to do the laundry is the tension caused by your child's disappointment or anger that her favorite shirt is dirty (still). At work you have to deal not only with the nagging discomfort that accompanies being behind schedule with assignments but also with the stress that accompanies your sense that you should be functioning better than you are.

The stress level is further raised by the negative effect of chronic fatigue on your mood, outlook, appetite, ability to think clearly, and memory. Perspective can be lost; the little bumps of normal daily life seem like mountains. You may forget to buy milk and then, because you are so tired, perceive your error as a catastrophe. And, since life goes on whether you are ready or not, you may find yourself, for the first time ever, unable to cope with serious issues or problems such as the loss of a loved one.

You may wish for a magic fairy to help you with your jobs and yet decline offers from willing friends, family, and co-workers. Why? Perhaps the accepting of help diminishes your sense of renewed control, freedom, and self-esteem. You feel stuck between what you want (independence, self-affirmation) and what you need (assistance, delayed gratification).

Unfairly, low energy carries the connotation of laziness for some people. You may decline help and push yourself beyond what common sense dictates in order to meet your own standards of performance. *You* may feel that you should be doing more and that you are lazy if you do not. Or you may worry that other people will interpret your complaints as malingering despite their show of understanding and support.

The problem is compounded by the common misconception that cancer brings a death sentence. Even though you are in remission, you sense that others perceive you as a doomed individual. You avoid anything that suggests illness, such as a needed nap, because of concern, justified or not, that others will see your napping as a sign of deterioration instead of as part of a normal recovery.

Studies have shown that people able to resume work after successful treatment perform at least as well as, and often better than, workers who have never been sick. However, in some circumstances survivors cannot resume prior jobs or responsibilities, temporarily or permanently. It may be unwise medically for a construction worker, an ice-skating instructor, or an orthopedic surgeon to resume work soon after bone marrow transplantation. However, they may try to return to work full-time anyway. By pushing themselves at work, they may feel that they can avoid facing their loss. They trade off the benefits of a reduced workload for the sense that they are back to normal and that nothing much has changed. And since there exists no blood test for measuring fatigue, it is hard for them and their doctors to know when they are ready to resume strenuous or stressful activities.

Another dimension to fatigue makes it challenging: how you look does not always reflect how you feel. If your skin turned purple (the deeper the purple, the more drained your energy), anyone who looked at you would know how you felt. And, unlike baldness or anemia, which goes away gradually and predictably, your energy level may fluctuate from hour to hour and day to day, making it difficult for you and those around you to predict how you will feel at any particular time. As it is, others can know whether you are fatigued, and how much, only if you tell them. This means dealing with repeated inquiries or providing a running report on your sense of well-being. Despite everyone's good intentions, this monitoring is itself tiresome.

Unlike baldness, vomiting, or pain, fatigue is not a dramatic or sympathy-engendering symptom. In our fast-paced society, "I'm tired" is a universal complaint. Generally speaking, treatment-related fatigue is more persistent and debilitating than that due to a busy lifestyle. It is alienating when healthy people respond to you by saying that they, too, are tired.

To make matters worse, fatigue is difficult to quantify. Under normal circumstances people use hyperbole to describe symptoms: "I'm completely exhausted. I'm dead tired." No useful words exist to communicate degrees of fatigue.

I believe that a new medical term is needed for the distinctive fatigue commonly seen after the completion of successful cancer treatment. I offer the term "postcancer fatigue" (PCF) as a handle for survivors, health care professionals, and caretakers trying to deal with this difficult problem. "Postcancer fatigue" captures the essence of this problem: not only that fatigue often persists after remission is achieved but that being tired is not just in one's head. Postcancer fatigue is a symptom that must be recognized and treated as such.

My hope is that, by describing and naming this condition, I will encourage a dialogue between clinicians and researchers, doctors and patients. Distinguishing this fatigue highlights the problem and will prevent underreporting by patients and undertreatment by the health care team. Patients will be reassured by this validation of their debility, and hope on their part will be nourished by the knowledge that research is being done to facilitate its prevention, detection, and treatment.

Precautions must be taken not to attribute someone's fatigue to postcancer fatigue before all known causes of fatigue have been ruled out or corrected. Even though the definition demands this, the desire to put a closure on your medical evaluation may induce you or your doctor to label your fatigue "postcancer fatigue" and end the evaluation prematurely.

Further research into postcancer fatigue—its incidence, its patterns of expression, its natural history, its relation to cancer recurrence and other medical problems, its cause, a marker (a specific and sensitive diagnostic test)—may suggest that it is actually part of a syndrome that occurs following treatment. Research is essential and may yield clues to as-yet-unanswered questions about cancer.

POSTCANCER FATIGUE (PCF)

The oncology literature acknowledges the existence of a characteristic fatigue that occurs following treatment when remission is achieved. It is not explained completely by detectable abnormalities and persists despite the evaluation and correction of all identifiable causes of fatigue. Anyone involved in the care of cancer survivors knows that fatigue is universal during and immediately following aggressive treatment and is difficult to understand, explain, or fix. Patients who experience postcancer fatigue describe it as different from any fatigue they ever experienced under healthy circumstances; they often describe it as feeling similar to infectious mononucleosis.

Postcancer fatigue is a symptom that

- is due to the effects of prior cancer and/or cancer treatment
- persists after all other known physical causes of fatigue have been ruled out or corrected
- persists after any depression, anxiety, or other emotional problem has been ruled out or resolved
- persists despite good-quality sleep, good nutrition, and abstinence from medicines that cause fatigue or sleepiness
- hinders the performance of activities of daily living (ADLs)

Postcancer fatigue affects daily life and requires significant adjustments in habits and schedules. If severe, it may prevent you from performing desired activities. Before your illness, when you felt wiped out, one or two good nights of sleep probably recharged your batteries and made you feel refreshed. With postcancer fatigue you may at times feel exhausted even after doing all the things that used to make you feel refreshed.

Before your illness you experienced a predictable pattern of progressive exhaustion after becoming sleep-deprived: you felt okay when you first got up, or after a cup or two of coffee, and then gradually got sleepy by late morning or early afternoon. Similarly, individuals with postcancer fatigue learn that their fatigue is worse under certain circumstances (before or after meals, before or after exercise, during and following family conflicts, before checkups, and so on) and that it worsens gradually. Diverse circumstances may exacerbate postcancer fatigue in different people.

Although some circumstances predictably make you feel worse, the pattern with postcancer fatigue is often variable, with days or weeks of more energy followed by days or weeks of extreme fatigue. In addition, people with this symptom often report episodic bouts of fatigue: they feel pretty good for a while, and then suddenly, while reading a book or working on a report, they are unexpectedly overwhelmed with debilitating fatigue. They may feel fine until halfway through lunch—and all at once become too tired to finish eating.

"Postcancer fatigue" is a term that can be applied only after all treatable causes of fatigue have been ruled out by your oncologist or internist, or have been corrected.

Is Postcancer Fatigue the Same As Chronic Fatigue or Chronic Fatigue Syndrome?

No. Postcancer fatigue is a symptom distinct from chronic fatigue and that seen in chronic fatigue syndrome. "Postcancer fatigue" applies only to weariness that occurs in people in remission following treatment, that is due to the prior cancer or its treatment, and that persists after all treatable causes of fatigue have been ruled out or been corrected.

In contrast, "chronic fatigue" is a term that describes a symptom but conveys nothing about its cause, course, or treatment. "Chronic fatigue syndrome," still a somewhat controversial concept, is defined not only by its unique symptom complex but also by the supposed causative agents, the usual course it takes, and the treatment.

What Causes Postcancer Fatigue?

Although the exact mechanism remains unknown, the scientific community accepts the view that residual effects of radiation, chemotherapy, or other cancer therapy can cause fatigue long after the completion of treatment. Since the definition of postcancer fatigue demands that all treatable causes of tiredness have been ruled out or corrected, as-yet-unidentified changes or abnormalities are the probable culprits. Three possible causes are

• the circulation of fatigue-causing substances released by dead, dying, or repairing cells

- changes in the parts of the brain that affect energy level, changes caused by prior cancer or treatment
- the residual inefficiency of otherwise normal cells and organs (e.g., muscles may appear normal on examination and with diagnostic tests but may be functioning subnormally as a result of changes on the cellular level, detectable only with sophisticated research technology)

Fatigue is a nonspecific symptom. It is difficult, if not impossible, to determine which of the hard-to-quantify possible causes are playing a role. You may have been treated optimally for depression; yet some residual refractory depression (depression unresponsive to treatment) persists. Or you may have a high risk of recurrent cancer, and chronic subclinical anxiety (it is present, but there is little sign of it) may be contributing to your fatigue. We need further study of the mechanisms of this symptom. The hope is that research will lead to effective means of prevention, detection, and treatment of postcancer fatigue.

Do All Cancer Survivors Get Postcancer Fatigue?

No. Survivors who required limited treatment usually recover fairly quickly and completely. Although some fatigue following treatment is almost universal, if it resolves after correction of an identified cause of fatigue, it was not postcancer fatigue.

One woman complained, "I'm running on empty, and I can't do what I need or want to do. It's making me feel depressed." An evaluation revealed iron deficiency anemia and low estrogen levels. She was placed on iron and estrogen replacement, and her fatigue and depression resolved completely over the subsequent month. She had anemia and reactive depression; she did not have postcancer fatigue.

Another woman with the same complaints and abnormalities (anemia and estrogen deficiency) was also treated with replacement iron and estrogen. After a few weeks she felt somewhat improved, but complained, "Now I'm running on an eighth of a tank all the time. I can get some stuff done, but if anything extra or stressful occurs, I can't handle it." After another year this, too, resolved. The medications took care of her anemia and estrogen deficiency, but not her postcancer fatigue.

How Long Does Postcancer Fatigue Last?

The same factors that affect the duration of fatigue in general would be expected to affect the duration of postcancer fatigue (see page 113). Anecdotal evidence suggests that for many survivors, it is a temporary, if protracted, condition. As a rule, the more intense and prolonged your treatment, the longer its aftereffects. As the population of survivors grows and research progresses, solid answers will become available.

What Can I Do If I Have Postcancer Fatigue?

Recognize that this is a real medical condition. Avoid blaming yourself with such thoughts as "I'm not trying hard enough. I must like being sick. My attitude isn't good enough." Avoid negative thoughts such as "If I'd known recovery was going to be so tough, I wouldn't have gone through the treatment. My doctors must have given me too much treatment; that's why I feel so awful." Postcancer fatigue is one of the aftereffects that requires patience and hopefulness.

The first step you need to take is getting evaluated for any treatable problem(s) that may be causing or exacerbating your malaise. Just as important, make sure that you are reevaluated periodically if your fatigue persists. Normal results obtained by an evaluation six or twelve months ago do not guarantee normal results now.

If your doctors have ruled out all other causes of fatigue, including recurrence, and conclude that you have postcancer fatigue, reassure yourself that nothing is being missed. Remind yourself that postcancer fatigue is real, is not due to any detectable (or treatable) problem, and is not just in your head. As long as you are reevaluated periodically, you can let go of the fear of recurrence or other medical problem between evaluations.

Find out what you can do to prevent any new medical problems or flare-ups of old ones. Conserve your physical and emotional energies. Doctors, nurses, social workers, psychologists, psychiatrists, and clergy can all help you find a balance between your energy needs and supplies. Adjusting to energy limitations may be a novelty for you, and it is not always obvious what the best way to pace yourself is.

Even when your fatigue is not *due* to emotional stress or problems, it can *cause* emotional and social stress. A healthy understanding of the problem and a healthy attitude toward it will help you cope with the necessary changes. Like your other losses, the losses accompanying postcancer fatigue (loss of energy, ability to do things, companionship, etc.) can be dealt with better when you accept emotional and spiritual support.

How Is Postcancer Fatigue Related to Depression?

As is discussed in the section on depression (pages 229–32), dealing with the consequences of postcancer fatigue can increase your risk of developing depression. Depression may have been ruled out when you were first evaluated, and you may be coping as well as humanly possible. You believe that you cannot always choose your circumstances, but you can choose how you deal with them. Yet, despite your positive attitude, wonderful support, and deep faith, the physical changes caused by the chronic stress of dealing with postcancer fatigue can increase the risk of becoming depressed.

Depression is usually associated with such symptoms as lack of interest in activities that usually bring pleasure, significant weight loss or gain, changed sleep patterns, decreased ability to concentrate, and morbid thoughts. However, depression can also manifest itself solely as fatigue. Treating the depression will take care of this fatigue.

When being evaluated for postcancer fatigue, you will be assessed for any component of depression that might benefit from counseling and/or medication. When depression is misdiagnosed as postcancer fatigue, you are denied the benefit of effective treatment.

Take steps to minimize the development of depression in the setting of postcancer fatigue:

• Learn about postcancer fatigue.
• Learn about energy conservation measures that will allow you to match your energy requirements to supplies.
• Learn to accept the changes and losses necessary to deal with your fatigue.
• Allow yourself to grieve the loss of energy.
• Develop new sources of enjoyment and relaxation to replace those no longer available. A variation of the same activity, such as playing competitive table tennis instead of full-court tennis, or working part-time instead of full-time, may help. On the other hand, this approach may be counterproductive because of the constant reminders of what has been lost. In this case an activity unlike the favored one is more therapeutic.

Postcancer fatigue is a medical problem like other medical problems. Proper evaluation and treatment allow you to minimize its effect on your new life.

What If My Doctors and Nurses Say There Is No Such Thing as Postcancer Fatigue?

Since "postcancer fatigue" is a newly coined term, time will tell whether it becomes widely accepted. However, no matter what it is called, the fatigue following cancer treatment is real. All of the information provided about the causes, course, evaluation, and treatment of postcancer fatigue applies to the cancer survivor with persistent fatigue after all treatable causes of fatigue are resolved. Work with your health care team to prevent, minimize, and treat all of your symptoms, including fatigue. Learn how to adjust so as to minimize the pain, debility, and loss following successful treatment.

PAIN

What If I Have Pain?

Pain is bodily distress. Aching joints, burning skin, cramped muscles, and knifelike chest twinges are sensations experienced as painful. Everyone feels pain in a unique way. One person may call an ambulance because of unbearable abdominal pain and be found to have a mildly inflamed appendix. Another person may walk into the emergency room complaining of moderate pain and be found to have a ruptured appendix with peritonitis.

Like fatigue, pain is a subjective symptom that is difficult to measure or quantify. It can fluctuate from hour to hour. Its effect on your daily life can range from being a mild nuisance to being the focus of your thoughts and actions. An understanding of the many factors that affect your experience of pain will help you prevent and control it.

Pain can be caused by physical changes due to your cancer or your treatments, such as

- a nerve damaged by cancer, chemotherapy, radiation, or surgery
- a broken bone
- blockage (of a blood vessel, a digestive tube, or the urinary tract)
- skin or bowel changes as a result of radiation
- infection
- swelling

The degree of your pain is influenced by such nonphysical factors as

- your anxiety and fear
- the meaning of your pain to you
- your sense of control over your pain
- your patterns of response to pain

How Does Pain Cause Anxiety?

Pain can generate concern about recurrent cancer or the development of a new medical problem. If you have completed therapy only recently, there has not been time to build up the experience of having pains that are unrelated to cancer or its treatments.

Pain can cause you to anticipate seeing a doctor. This anticipation can evoke many of the anxieties seen in "checkup anxiety" (see pages 236–38).

Many people have the misconception that cancer is usually a painful disease. When pain develops for whatever reason, you may fear that the pain is due to cancer and is the harbinger of greater pain. Many times this thought process works at a subconscious level.

How Does Anxiety Affect Pain?

Anxiety and pain feed each other in a vicious cycle. If your pain causes you to feel anxious, this anxiety can increase your perception of the pain; this increased perception of pain can cause increased anxiety; and so on.

Anxiety alone can create pain. Anxiety and uncertainty about your health may lead you to such a degree of self-monitoring that you are aware of every little change or sensation. Under normal circumstances a minor symptom would be noticed and then ignored, or not even perceived in the first place. Under circumstances of intense self-vigilance a minor symptom tends to be detected and even amplified. Anxiety about its significance and fear of progressive pain will increase both your anxiety and your level of pain.

If you have no medical problems with swallowing and no symptoms related to swallowing, try this simple experiment to demonstrate how pain and anxiety are related: pay attention to your swallowing for the next two minutes. Swallowing your saliva triggers a sequence of muscle contractions in the esophagus. If you pay attention to your normal swallowing, you become aware of sensations that are normally ignored. Intense concentration may even make it more difficult deliberately to initiate a swallow.

Simply paying attention to your body has altered your perception and created a symptom (difficulty in swallowing). Now, to take this experiment one step further, imagine that you are worried that your difficulty in swallowing saliva can mean that you have a serious medical problem. Anxiety about what your symptom means, added to your already heightened awareness of the symptom, magnifies your perception of the symptom and your anxiety level.

Just as your attention to and anxiety about a symptom can amplify your symptom and anxiety, your learning to distract yourself from the symptom and decrease your anxiety can bring relief. After cancer, symptom management includes breaking the vicious cycle of anxiety–pain.

Obviously, this approach is applicable only in the management of pain or symptoms that are not new and that have been properly evaluated. Your anxiety about a symptom is valuable in getting your attention and pushing you to have the symptom evaluated. Once you have done that, the anxiety is no longer serving a beneficial function and becomes counterproductive.

Anxiety is beneficial when it helps you do the right things. It is counterproductive if it persists after you do all the right things to take care of the anxiety-provoking problem.

What Makes Pain Worse?

Depending on the physical cause of the pain, factors that can affect the type or amount of pain you experience include

- activities such as walking, maintaining a certain position, or eating certain foods
- weather conditions
- bowel or bladder function
- hormonal balance
- fatigue
- anxiety
- sleep deprivation
- depression
- deconditioning
- malnutrition

What Can I Do, If I Have Pain, to Help Relieve It?

Enormous progress has been made in understanding and relieving acute and chronic pain due to noncancerous conditions. Many of the approaches are applicable to pain due to cancer or its treatment. A vital starting point is to get the facts about the source of your pain. Find out whether anything can be done with medicine, surgery, or other therapy that can correct the physical problems that are causing your pain. While your pain is being evaluated, and certainly after its cause has been identified, take steps to get the pain under control.

Work with your doctors to find the safest medicine for relieving your pain. In most cases, it is best to take your pain medicine around the clock until you are consistently pain-free. Studies have documented that people in pain who take pain medicine only "as needed" require more total medication and experience less satisfactory pain control than people who are taking regularly scheduled pain medicine. With the pain under better control, you can work with your doctor on physical activities that may help alleviate the pain.

Many people with uncontrolled pain develop poor physical habits that cause additional problems. For instance, favoring a painful arm can cause secondary weakness and stiffness in the limb. Uncontrolled pain also leads to poor psychological habits. If chronic pain leads you to avoid outings and social contact, you deprive yourself of the companionship and distraction that are so valuable in the transition to your new life after cancer.

The chief function of pain is to draw attention to a problem so that you can take measures to fix it. Nothing is gained and much is lost by enduring pain without investigating its source, or after having the source explained. Many physical and behavioral postures that reduce pain may prolong its duration, prevent healing, and cause further problems.

Your mind possesses the power to help diminish your sensation of pain. Learn about biofeedback and relaxation techniques. Effective relaxation will reduce pain caused by muscle spasm affecting the injured organ. In addition, a state of relaxation will so diminish the perception of pain that the pain, even if unchanged, becomes more tolerable. Learn how to divert your attention away from your pain. The more you focus on your pain and the more you arrange your life around your pain, the more your pain will have control over you.

Your mind can help through rational problem solving. Evaluate how your pain is affecting your activities and your interactions with other people. Find a way to get around the limits currently imposed by your pain so that you can resume your activities and normalize your interactions. You may need outside help to figure out ways to compensate for limitations, such as that offered by occupational therapists, physical therapists, physiotherapists, orthopedists, and support groups.

One woman loved her weekly evening bridge game. After completing her cancer treatment, she experienced joint stiffness and pain that were worse in the evenings. She shared her problem with her game partners. For the next few months they played in the morning. Instead of sacrificing a source of enjoyment, distraction, and fellowship, they made changes to accommodate her problem.

Many hurdles are not so easily overcome. One barber found it painful to stand for any length of time after his treatments were completed. At first he handled the pain stoically but was physically and emotionally miserable by the end of the day. Pain medication made him too sleepy to work. A social worker referred him to someone who found a special chair that enabled him to be seated for most of the hair cutting. His recovery was enhanced by the benefits of good pain control, good back support, and the emotional lift he felt from getting back to work.

Take steps to control your pain. Beliefs, expectations, and will power play a major role in pain control.

Learn to control your pain so that your pain does not control you.

What Is the Goal of Pain Treatment?

The goal of pain management is to make your pain manageable so that you can continue your life in a meaningful way.

Optimal pain management means minimizing physical pain and minimizing any adverse response to or consequence of the pain.

In some cases, it means learning how to accept a certain level of pain and making adjustments in your lifestyle.

How Does Self-relaxation Work to Relieve Pain?

When you learn self-relaxation or meditation, you learn to focus on something, such as a mental image of a calm lake, to distract you from pain signals. Through various techniques, you can learn to decrease tension in your muscles. This allows you to achieve a state of deep relaxation that provides immediate comfort and helps replenish your physical and emotional energy stores.

How can focusing on something stop you from feeling pain? Your perception of pain is affected by your attention to it. For example, an ice skater who sustains a gash during competition may be unaware of the cut until the performance is completed and the dripping blood is noticed. This same skater might scream with pain when receiving a routine vaccination. Or, while reading an exciting book, you may not notice the sound of the bathtub over-flowing in the next room. And yet, at night you may be unable to sleep because of the sound of a dripping faucet. Although you cannot always control the source of pain, you can control your attention to it.

Studies are in progress to determine whether regular relaxation measurably improves the immune system and prevents medical problems, such as heart disease and cancer.

You can learn relaxation techniques from qualified counselors and psychiatrists. There are also books, pamphlets, and audio-tapes on self-relaxation and meditation. Information and tapes are available from the Stress/Health Management Center, 621 Mary-land Avenue, NE, Washington, DC.

How Does Biofeedback Work to Relieve Pain?

Biofeedback works on the principle that if you have information (feedback) on how close you are to your goal, you can make adjustments to get closer to the goal. A baseball pitcher gets feed-back about each pitch from the umpire (low and outside, strike, and so on) and is thus able to make adjustments in the next pitch. When you are trying to lose weight, you step on a scale to get feedback (your weight) in order to adjust your diet and exercise.

At times it is helpful to be able to control bodily functions such as muscle tension. Muscle tension can cause severe headaches or can increase pain near a surgical site. Muscle tension is not something that you can easily measure just by looking at or feeling your muscle. Biofeedback is a technique that overcomes the limits of your senses by using a machine to give you information about your muscle tension in a signal that is easy for you to measure. Sensors attached to your shoulders, for example, measure the tension in the underlying muscles. The measurement of muscle tension is converted to a signal such as sound, light, or a line on a graph. As your muscle tension gets higher, the sound gets louder, the light gets brighter, or the line goes higher on the graph. You use this information to learn how to reduce your muscle tension. With time and practice, you can learn how to respond to the subtle information from your leg muscles on your own, without the amplification provided by the biofeedback equipment.

Biofeedback has been used successfully for years to control many types of headache, irritable bowel, high and low blood pressure, seizures, muscle weakness, and circulation problems.

Since the physical changes that accompany stress can worsen your pain and your perception of it, learning to counteract your body's stress response is helpful. Biofeedback can help you recognize and counteract your physical responses to stress and anxiety.

For example, one woman had bone pain in her leg after her cancer surgery. Whenever her bone hurt, she became anxious that her cancer was back. Her anxiety would cause her to tense her leg muscles unconsciously, which would cause her pain to increase. By learning to relax her muscles through biofeedback, she decreased her pain significantly without adding pain medicines. Relaxing her muscles also helped her block the vicious pain–anxiety–pain cycle without resorting to tranquilizers.

Is It Important to Treat Chronic Mild Pain?

It is vital that chronic pain be evaluated and treated. Most people can withstand severe pain for a short while, especially if they know that it will end. The effect of chronic pain is different from that of acute (short-term) pain. Even mild pain depletes your physical and emotional reserves and can cause you to feel tired, irritable, and depressed. Sleep can be disturbed, which often intensifies your perception of pain. Pain extracts a psychological toll by reminding you of your cancer experience, keeping your fears and anxieties close to the surface, and making it more difficult for you to deal with everything.

Is Pain Ever Expected after Cancer Treatment?

Many conditions (such as a bone fracture) and treatments (such as surgery) are expected to cause pain. However, just because pain is an expected normal aftereffect it does not mean it should go untreated. Pain should be evaluated thoroughly, its cause determined, and the best treatment found. Medications can be prescribed when indicated. Nonpharmacological measures for pain control can be pursued.

If I Have Pain, Do I Have to Report It at My Checkups?

Absolutely. Pain is a subjective phenomenon. Your doctor will *not* know how much pain you have by your exam or test results. Your doctor can assess and treat your pain only if you tell him or her about it.

A retired teacher presented herself graciously at her checkups. Well groomed and always smiling, she focused on her progress. Her doctor, satisfied with her normal exam and test results, reassured her that she was indeed doing beautifully. She never gave her doctor a clue that she had nighttime pain that interfered with sleep and fed her unvoiced anxiety. It was only when the woman's daughter called the doctor to discuss the problem that it was addressed.

Your doctors can help you with a problem only if you tell them about it.

SLEEP

What If I Have Trouble Sleeping?

Sleep is a state of relaxation that restores your physical and emotional energies. Regular sleep is vital in order for you to function normally while awake. After cancer your usual sleep patterns can be upset by

- medications
- emotional stress, anxiety, or depression
- change in your daily schedule
- pain

Good-quality sleep is an important ingredient in recovery. Make changes to encourage regular, good-quality sleep, even if it means taking medication for a while. You can do many things to facilitate good sleep:

- Adjust the timing, dose, or choice of medications that may be keeping you awake, such as decongestants and other cold remedies or steroids.
- Eliminate dietary stimulants such as caffeine in coffee, tea, chocolate, colas, and certain over-the-counter pain medications. This is especially important in the afternoon and evening.
- Avoid long afternoon naps, which may make it hard to fall asleep at night.
- Do something relaxing to get ready for sleep.
- Arrange your pain medication schedule to control pain when you go to sleep.

• Avoid alcohol at bedtime (it may help you fall asleep but will impair the quality and duration of sleep).

What About Nightmares?

Nightmares, distressing dreams, occur irregularly throughout life. During periods of emotional tension, you may notice an increase in the frequency, vividness, or daytime recall of your nightmares. After cancer this can be related to

- your medications
- uncontrolled pain
- posttraumatic stress (emotional stress following a traumatic event or experience)

Nightmares tend to become more frequent after one's survival of any traumatic experience. Now that your treatments are over, your subconscious is processing what you went through. Some of your surfacing fears and anxieties may express themselves in nightmares. Remember that they are just dreams, not reality. Nightmares do not predict the future or cause events to occur. If they are persistent or anxiety producing, discuss them with your doctor.

AFTEREFFECTS INVOLVING THE NERVOUS SYSTEM

What Causes Numbness?

Numbness, or other change in your sensation of touch, can be due to a

- medication effect
- cancer effect
- nerve injury from the cancer or surgery
- vitamin deficiency

Does Numbness Go Away?

If the numbness is caused by drugs, it will often slowly reverse after the drug is stopped. If caused by a vitamin deficiency, it may reverse with vitamin replacement. If caused by nerve injury from the cancer or surgery, it may or may not reverse. Injured nerves take months to years to repair themselves. Even reversible nerve injuries are notorious for taking a long time to improve or resolve.

What Causes Headaches?

Headaches may be due to

- side effects of current medication
- muscle tension
- hormonal changes
- sinus problems, such as allergies
- eyestrain
- emotional stress
- brain metastases

If I Feel an Electric Shock When I Bend My Head Forward, What Should I Do?

A small percentage of people develop Lhermitte's sign after radiation to certain areas of the chest (e.g., after mantle radiation given for Hodgkin's disease). It usually begins six weeks to three months after completion of the radiation and resolves by itself over time. This self-limited cause of electric shock sensation must be distinguished by your doctor from more serious causes.

What If My Vision Is Different?

Vision can be affected by

- side effects of current medications
- temporary or permanent effects of cancer therapy

• temporary or permanent effects of your cancer
• normal age-related changes

Notify your oncologist of the vision change. Have an opthalmologist evaluate you for eye problems or the need for new eyeglasses.

What If My Hearing Is Worse?

Decreased hearing can be due to

• side effects of current medications
• late effects of certain antibiotics
• temporary or permanent effects of cancer therapy
• temporary or permanent effects of your cancer
• age-related changes in your ears

Have your ears checked by an otolaryngologist (ENT doctor) in order to

• document your current auditory acuity (hearing ability)
• fix any easily treatable problems, such as wax or fluid buildup
• assess your need for a hearing aid

What Does It Mean If My Thinking Is Less Clear Than before My Cancer?

Clouded thinking, frequent loss of train of thought, or difficulty in processing or remembering things is a common problem after cancer treatment. One young accountant found it hard to remember telephone numbers and calculate figures in his head. Working with numbers had formerly been his claim to fame. He was afraid that he had survived his cancer only to develop Alzheimer's disease.

Changes in memory and mental clarity are distressing. You may feel diminished self-esteem. Your awareness that you are different from the way you were is intensified. You may get anxious that something is seriously wrong with you.

On a practical level the mental changes affect the quality and efficiency of your work. This can cause increased stress at home and at work. Forgetting to pay the rent, pick up the children from camp, or take out the garbage on pickup day disrupts everyone's day. When you are aware of the mental changes, you may try to compensate by concentrating hard on everything you do, leaving extra time for "goofs," double-checking everything you do. Such efforts will help you perform normally but will drain your energy.

Tell your doctor if you notice changes in your memory or your ability to think clearly. The changes have many possible physical or emotional explanations. After evaluating you, your doctor may be able to reassure you that there is nothing seriously wrong and that you can expect the changes to resolve with time. This news will save you a lot of worry (about recurrent cancer, say, or swelling in the brain). If something needs medical attention, it will be attended to sooner rather than later.

Many medical and emotional changes after treatment can affect memory and cause clouded thinking. Any combination of the following may be playing a role:

- side effects of current medications
- aftereffects of cancer treatment
- aftereffects of your cancer (e.g., brain cancer)
- hormonal imbalance
- fatigue
- emotional stress, anxiety, or depression

What If My Balance Is Off?

A sense of imbalance or vertigo can be due to

- side effects of current medications
- aftereffects of cancer treatments

• aftereffects of your cancer (e.g., a tumor of the brain or ear)
• allergies
• hormonal imbalance

AFTEREFFECTS INVOLVING THE CIRCULATION SYSTEM

What If I Have Swelling?

Generalized swelling (swelling all over) or leg swelling can be due to

• medication effect
• hormonal effect
• poor circulation in veins
• weak kidneys
• heart problems
• liver problems

Swelling in a small area or in one arm or leg can be due to

• damage or blockage to the lymph system of the area
• blockage of a vein
• other local problems

Your doctor can tell you whether

• your swelling indicates a significant problem in important organs, such as your heart or kidneys, or is basically a cosmetic issue
• your swelling is expected to be temporary or permanent
• there are medicines or other measures you can take to relieve the swelling safely

You need to notify your doctor if the swelling is new or if fever, pain, tenderness, redness, heat, or overlying skin changes in the swollen area develop.

What Does It Mean If I Often Faint?

Problems that can cause you to feel faint include

- anemia
- deconditioning (the loss of normal strength and tone in muscles and blood vessels because of reduced exercise and activity)
- damage to the nervous system
- heart rhythm problems
- hormonal imbalance

Am I at Increased Risk of Heart Problems?

Certain cancer treatments carry some risk of heart injury:

- high-dose Adriamycin—risk is directly related to the total dose of Adriamycin received over your lifetime
- high-dose radiation to the chest

How Do I Know Whether I Have Heart Problems?

Call your doctor if you develop

- shortness of breath
- chest heaviness, tightness, squeezing, or pain
- chest heaviness or shortness of breath with exertion, such as walking up stairs or lifting groceries
- swelling in your feet and legs
- fever
- light-headedness
- loss of consciousness, no matter how brief
- palpitations (abnormally rapid throbbing or fluttering of the heart)

AFTEREFFECTS INVOLVING THE GASTROINTESTINAL SYSTEM

What If My Appetite Is Still Poor?

All the factors that affect appetite during cancer treatment can continue to affect it after treatment is completed, such as

- medications
- changes in the digestive system due to the cancer
- changes in the digestive system due to the treatments
- weakness
- infections
- impaired or altered sense of taste or smell
- depression and emotional stress

If My Appetite Is Poor, When Will It Return to Normal?

It can take many months for your appetite to return. You must take steps to evaluate your lack of appetite if

- you are not able to eat enough for healing
- you are losing weight or getting weaker
- you have pain in your mouth, throat, esophagus, stomach, or rectum
- you have difficulty swallowing
- your stools are black, maroon, or bloody

What If It Hurts to Swallow?

Changes that make swallowing difficult or painful include

- irritation of the esophagus from radiation, chemotherapy, or acid reflux from the stomach
- infection of the esophagus, such as viral or fungal infections
- decreased saliva

• narrowing of the esophagus
• spasm of the muscles of the esophagus

What Is a Stricture of the Esophagus?

Months to years following radiation to the chest, some patients develop scarring of the esophagus that causes the opening to be narrowed. This narrowing, or stricture, makes it difficult to swallow solids. The narrowed esophagus can be dilated, or stretched, fairly easily.

If I Have Diarrhea, What Is Causing It?

Diarrhea can be due to

• medications
• inadequate dietary fiber
• changes in your diet
• radiation changes to the digestive tract
• chemotherapy-related changes in the intestines or colon that cause poor absorption of food
• cancer-related changes in the intestines or colon that cause poor absorption
• shortened intestines from surgery
• infection in the digestive tract
• lactose (milk sugar) intolerance

If I Have Diarrhea, What Can I Do for It?

Your doctor has to determine why you have the diarrhea in order to advise treatment. If it is due to medication, your doctor may change your medication and/or add dietary fiber. If it is due to radiation changes, dietary changes and/or antidiarrhea medications may help. If diarrhea is due to infection, you may need antibiotics.

What Causes Constipation?

Constipation can be caused by

- medications, such as pain medications
- inadequate fluids in diet
- inadequate dietary fiber
- damage to the nervous system affecting the gut
- inactivity
- obstruction (blockage) of the lower gastrointestinal tract by a scar

What Can Be Done about Constipation?

Talk with your doctor about

- stool softeners
- increased oral fluids
- dietary fiber, if there is no contraindication
- increased activity

AFTEREFFECTS INVOLVING THE ENDOCRINE SYSTEM (HORMONES)

Am I at Risk for Low Thyroid (Hypothyroidism)?

Hypothyroidism is a fairly common medical condition independently of cancer. Your routine comprehensive exam by your internist or general practitioner includes evaluation of your thyroid. You are at an increased risk for developing low thyroid if you

- received radiation to the neck
- received radiation or surgery to the pituitary
- are on interferon
- are over fifty

If I Have Diabetes, and It Has Gotten out of Control, Why?

Diabetes can be affected adversely by

- weight gain or weight loss
- changes in absorption of food
- changes in absorption of diabetes medicine
- effects of cancer or cancer therapy
- effects of medications, such as steroids

Am I at Increased Risk for Developing Diabetes?

Your general medical exam includes an evaluation for diabetes. Diabetes is a common disease independently of cancer. Your treatment may have had no effect on your risk of developing diabetes, and you will or will not develop diabetes just as if you had never had cancer. On the other hand, your cancer treatment may have caused changes in your body that cause you to develop diabetes sooner than you would have otherwise.

Some people develop diabetes, temporarily or permanently, from their treatment, people who probably would never have developed diabetes otherwise. Your doctor can tell you whether any of your treatments increased your chance of developing diabetes.

What Are Symptoms of Diabetes?

Diabetes is marked by a loss of normal control of blood sugar. High blood sugar can cause such symptoms as

- increased thirst
- increased urination
- increased appetite
- weight loss
- blurred vision
- poor wound healing

AFTEREFFECTS INVOLVING THE REPRODUCTIVE AND SEXUAL FUNCTIONS

What If My Sexual Drive Is Diminished or Absent?

Unlike that of animals, whose sexuality is fairly well programmed, your sexual drive is affected by your body, your emotional state, your relationship with your partner, and the stresses in your life. Sexual dysfunction, especially if it has appeared only since your cancer diagnosis, is a symptom that suggests medical, emotional, and/or social problems.

Many people report diminished or absent libido, or sexual drive, after completion of cancer treatment. In some cases, it is directly related to your cancer or its treatment. It may be the result of, for example,

- brain surgery that affected the part of the brain dealing with libido
- medicine that blocks hormones that contribute to libido

Decreased libido can be indirectly related to your cancer and its treatment. It can be a manifestation of

- fatigue
- medication effect
- pain
- depression
- emotional stress or anxiety about yourself
- poor self-image or fear of rejection
- strained relationship with your sexual partner

Focusing attention on sexual difficulties will encourage you to identify and attend to problems that can be solved or reduced. Working through the sensitive issues of sexual dysfunction can foster emotional closeness with your sexual partner that will spill over into other spheres of your life together.

What Can Be Done about a Diminished Sexual Drive?

Work with your doctors to find out why your drive is diminished. They can determine whether medical problems are contributing to the change. If medications may be playing a role, discuss the possibility of using alternative medicines that have less effect on libido.

If there are no obvious medical abnormalities, or if medical problems are permanent, evaluate your general level of energy and your mood. If you are fatigued, make efforts to get more rest. If you are anxious or depressed, try to deal with the sources of these feelings as well as the feelings themselves. Sometimes an alleviation of fatigue, anxiety, and depression suffices to lessen sexual difficulties. Even if medication or a medical problem is causing or contributing to the sexual problem, attention to your energy and mood will help.

It is common to have an altered body image, either because of obvious changes such as the loss of a body part or the placement of a stoma (opening for a "bag" to collect urine or feces) or because of general associations with having cancer. Addressing the issue of body image and self-confidence will encourage improved self-esteem and a return to healthy sexual function.

If you had a problem with self-image before your cancer, this is a good opportunity to deal with it. Open discussion is an effective means of moving toward resolving problems of self-esteem. Try talking with

- your sexual partner
- a social worker, professional counselor, or therapist with a special interest in sexuality
- other cancer survivors of the same kind of cancer or same kind of surgery

Decreased sexual desire can reflect a change in your relationship to your sexual partner. Human sexual desire and function are affected by feelings of anger, disappointment, fear of rejection, and frustration with the sexual partner, as well as by feelings of inadequacy.

Occasionally, patients or their partners may be sexually inhibited by concerns that

- cancer is infectious or contagious (it is *not* contagious)
- sexual activity may weaken or hurt the recovering partner
- the cancer is a punishment for prior "bad behavior" (this may be a conscious or a subconscious thought)

Decreased sexual interest is a normal part of grieving and spontaneously returns to normal with time. If you are sad about personal losses, others' losses, or the general pain and losses of life, you will have to start to grieve these losses before your sexual desire returns.

(for men) What Causes Impotence?

Impotence is the inability of a man to achieve and maintain an erection. It can be temporary or permanent, partial or complete. Things that affect sexual function include

- damage to nerves of the sexual organs
- damage to vessels of sexual organs
- damage to the sexual organs
- depression or grief
- side effect of current medications
- aftereffect of cancer medications
- fatigue
- anxiety, depression, or emotional stress
- change in emotional relationship with sexual partner
- pain

(for women) What Causes Decreased Lubrication? Decrease or Loss of Orgasm?

Lubrication and orgasm can be affected by

- hormonal changes
- medication
- damage to nerves to genitals from surgery or radiation
- damage to lining of female genital tract from chemotherapy
- damage to lining of female genital tract from local radiation
- genital infection
- depression, grief, anxiety, or emotional stress
- change in emotional relationship with sexual partner
- pain

If I Have Experienced a Change in My Sexual Functioning, What Can I Do?

Do not assume that sexual difficulties are due to an emotional problem. Discuss with your oncologist the changes you have noticed. Find out whether your cancer or its treatment could have played a role in the change in your sexual function. Ask whether you can expect your problems to resolve by themselves and how quickly you can expect to see a difference. Learn about everything you can do to help your sexual function recover.

Treatment options include

- medications
- surgery
- individual counseling
- support groups or group counseling
- family or couple counseling
- behavioral therapy

What If I Am Reluctant to Talk about My Sexual Function with My Oncologist?

Many people are reluctant to mention sexual concerns to their oncologists. This may be because you

- are embarrassed or ashamed of your loss of sexual function
- see your oncologist as someone who deals with life-and-death decisions, making your concern about sexual function appear petty
- are grateful to have survived and do not want to appear ungrateful by complaining
- do not want to deal with any more medical issues

Your ability to function sexually at a level that is satisfactory to you and your partner is an important factor in your overall quality of life.

What If I Have Tried to Talk with My Oncologist about Sexual Difficulties But Obtained No Satisfactory Answers or Advice?

If you tried to communicate your concerns about sexual function but were too uncomfortable to deal with it or if your doctor seemed uncomfortable or unable to deal with the topic, look for help elsewhere. Professionals who are well trained and comfortable dealing with issues of sexuality include

- gynecologists
- urologists
- psychologists specializing in sexual dysfunction

You can obtain a referral to a sex counselor with experience in the problems resulting from physical illness by writing or calling the American Association of Sex Educators, Counselors and Therapists, 435 N. Michigan Avenue, Suite 1717, Chicago, IL 60611, 312-644-0828.

(for men) Has My Treatment Affected My Ability to Father Children?

Radiation therapy to the testicles can cause sterility. Whether or not it is permanent depends on

- your age when treated
- the total dose of radiation received
- use of concomitant chemotherapy

Chemotherapy can also cause temporary or permanent sterility. Sterility is the more likely and has a greater chance of being permanent,

- the older you are when treated
- the higher the total dose of chemotherapeutic agents known to cause sterility
- the longer the duration of exposure to chemotherapeutic agents known to cause sterility
- the larger the number of drugs used that are known to cause sterility

Is Posttreatment Sterility Ever Reversible?

Yes. Men and women have been known to regain fertility twelve to sixty months following completion of cancer treatment.

Does My Exposure to Radiation and/or Chemotherapy Increase the Risk of Congenital Abnormalities in My Children Conceived in the Future?

Most studies addressing this issue have failed to show an increased incidence of congenital malformations when the mother or father was previously treated for cancer. The conclusions are somewhat limited by the relatively small number of babies born to cancer survivors (although this number is increasing annually) and by the fact that most analyses are based on data for survivors of Hodgkin's disease (a type of lymphoma).

There is some evidence to suggest that women previously treated with chemotherapy and/or radiation who are now fertile have a higher incidence of miscarriage.

Cancer survivors of both sexes who are contemplating pregnancy should strongly consider getting genetic counseling. In this cutting-edge field of medicine, experts in genetic counseling are best equipped to help you make an informed decision with the information available.

(for men) When Can I Think about Safely Fathering a Child?

Discuss with your oncologist your desires, needs, and concerns regarding conception. In general, you will need to wait until the quality and counts of your sperm appear satisfactory. Wait until you feel ready for the stress of a new baby emotionally, physically, and financially. Recovery from cancer entails a stressful transition, and you should take on additional major stresses only after weighing the pros and cons, and the risks and benefits to everyone involved.

(for women) When Can I Think about Becoming Pregnant?

Discuss with your doctor

- when you are felt to be adequately recovered to carry a full-term pregnancy
- when your cancer situation is felt not to be jeopardized by the normal changes of pregnancy, such as the hormonal changes
- when your cancer situation will no longer require tests that would put a fetus at risk, such as X rays or scans

When possible, wait until you feel ready to handle the physical, emotional, and financial stress of a new baby.

What Are My Options for Becoming Pregnant If My Cancer Treatment Has Permanently Decreased My Fertility (Made Me Subfertile) or Made Me Permanently Sterile?

Various options are available for women rendered subfertile or sterile by their cancer treatment. For example, some women are candidates for ovum donation (implantation of an egg from a donor). If childbearing is an issue, seek consultation with specialists in assisted reproductive techniques. The names of doctors who work in this high-tech specialty can be obtained from the ob-gyn department of your local hospital or from the American Fertility Society, 1209 Montgomery Highway, Birmingham, AL 35216-2809, 205-978-5000. You should review with your oncologist any decisions regarding treatment for fertility before you proceed. The potential for problems or risks in your specific case as a result of proposed treatments must be considered.

What Does It Mean If My Periods Have Stopped?

Periods may become irregular or stop altogether if your cancer or its treatment has affected the delicate balance of hormones that governs the normal menstrual cycle. Many other conditions cause cessation of periods. Notify your doctor if your periods change or stop.

If My Periods Have Stopped, Will They Start Up Again?

Your periods may start up again depending on

- your age when you received cancer treatment
- the type of treatment received
- the dose and duration of treatment

If I Am Not Having Periods, Can I Get Pregnant?

Yes. Although very unlikely, it is still possible that your normal cycle will return. If you are not using contraception, you risk getting pregnant before your first period.

If I Am Having Periods, Can I Assume That I Am Fertile?

No. There are many factors that govern fertility. You can have periods without eggs' being released for fertilization.

Are There Any Problems Associated with Not Having Periods?

Women stop having periods at menopause. When menopause occurs at any earlier-than-average age for whatever reason (such as surgical removal of the ovaries, chemotherapy- or radiation therapy–related loss of ovarian function, or a familial tendency), the woman is said to have premature menopause, or early menopause.

The hormonal changes of menopause are felt to be related to the development of thinning of the bones (osteoporosis) and the development of coronary artery disease (which can cause a heart attack) in women at risk. The earlier the age at menopause, the higher the risk of these problems. Menopausal women can pursue a number of measures to offset the changes of menopause. Discuss with your doctor your treatment options. When any doctor discusses estrogen replacement therapy (ERT), be sure you understand the pros and cons of such therapy in your particular case regarding

- your risk of recurrent cancer
- your risk of a new cancer
- the role of ERT in prevention of osteoporosis
- the role of ERT in prevention of heart disease
- your risk of blood clots
- the treatment of menopausal symptoms

Some women find menopause liberating and its side effects minimal. Others find that it requires a physically and/or emotionally very difficult adjustment. Seek information and support if your menopause is difficult.

AFTEREFFECTS INVOLVING THE SKIN

How Does Chemotherapy Affect the Skin?

Chemotherapy can affect the skin by

- causing direct changes in the skin cells
- causing changes to blood vessels under the skin
- exacerbating preexisting skin conditions
- allowing skin infections to develop that are normally prevented by a healthy immune system

How Does Radiation Affect the Skin?

Radiation can affect the skin by

- causing changes to exposed skin
- causing changes to the blood vessels under the skin

If I Have Skin Changes from My Radiation, How Long Will They Last?

Skin changes that can occur during and soon after radiation include

- redness
- sensitivity or discomfort
- warmth
- blisters
- skin breakdown

How long the skin changes last will depend on

- the area radiated (the back, the armpit, the groin, and the hands are more sensitive to the changes of radiation)
- the total dose of radiation received
- the type of radiation received
- previous surgery or concomitant chemotherapy
- infection

What Are Late Skin Changes of Radiation?

Changes in the skin that occur months to years following radiation include

- thinning of the skin
- contracture (tightening) of the skin
- telangiectasia (tiny red blood vessels seen on the skin)
- darkening or lightening compared to nonradiated skin
- problem with trauma-induced bruising or tearing
- slower, poorer healing after surgery or cuts

What If My Skin Is Dry?

After cancer therapy your skin may be dry because of

- injury, permanent or temporary, to the oil apparatus of the skin
- sensitivity to drying agents (water, soaps)

What Is Radiation Recall?

Radiation can cause permanent, if invisible, changes in the radiated skin, such that when you receive chemotherapy the area of skin previously radiated develops a reaction. If you received radiation to your shoulder, and years from now you took chemotherapy, you would have a chance of developing a reaction in the skin overlying your shoulder. This would depend on how much radiation you received, the chemotherapeutic agents used, and other factors, as yet unclear.

What If My Skin Is Sensitive to Light?

Your skin may be extra sensitive to light because

- some chemotherapy causes sun sensitivity that lasts for a few weeks to months after completion of the therapy
- some medications, such as certain antibiotics, cause sun sensitivity
- radiated skin can become extra sensitive to the damaging effects of the sun

What If I Get Many Rashes Now, Although I Never Had Rashes Before?

You may tend to get rashes because of

- current medications
- changes in your immune system from your cancer or cancer treatments that make you react to yourself
- changes in your immune system from your cancer or cancer treatment that make you more sensitive to external agents
- emotional nervousness

What Can Cause Skin to Change Color?

Your skin may appear to have a different hue because of

- medication effects
- effects of change in diet
- effects of certain vitamins
- hormonal changes
- radiation effects to exposed area

What If Little Cuts and Bumps Take Long to Heal?

If your skin is more fragile, you may bruise or cut yourself more easily. Bruises and cuts may take longer to heal because of residual changes in your immune system that take months to normalize. In some cases, you are healing as fast as you did before your treatments, but you are more sensitive to changes in your body. Close monitoring of your cuts and bumps makes the healing process seem slow ("A watched pot never boils").

Do I Need to Take Any Special Precautions with My Skin?

There are steps all people should take to protect their skin, whether or not they have ever had cancer. They are especially important after radiation to sun-exposed areas of your body or if you notice that your skin is drier or more sensitive to sunlight. These steps include

- avoiding sun exposure, especially between 10 A.M. and 2 P.M.
- avoiding tanning booths
- using sunscreen regularly (SPF at least 15)
- avoiding drying agents
- using moisturizers liberally
- avoiding harsh rubbing
- making sure a skin exam is done periodically as part of your routine medical examinations
- monitoring your skin for spots or moles that change (become itchy, develop an irregular border, bleed, change color)

What Is Shingles?

Shingles is a skin eruption caused by reactivation of the dormant chicken pox virus, herpes zoster. Shingles usually begins as burning or pain in a strip of skin, which is followed by the eruption of groups of vesicles (blisters) or pustules (pimples) in the distribution of the nerve involved. Occasionally, but not commonly, the virus can spread widely in the body from the nerve.

Who Gets Shingles?

Anyone can get shingles, but it is uncommon in healthy people under fifty years old. Radiation therapy, chemotherapy, and suppression of the immune system are all thought to allow reactivation of the virus. It is not uncommon to have a bout of shingles in the first two years after treatment for Hodgkin's disease. It is often seen in AIDS patients.

What Should I Do If I Think I Might Have Shingles?

Call your doctor immediately, and specify that you are concerned about shingles. Antiviral therapy is available that, if administered early, can

- shorten the course of skin eruption
- bring about earlier relief of symptoms

Your doctor may feel comfortable making the diagnosis over the telephone on the basis of your description. Many times your doctor will need to see the rash to confirm the diagnosis.

When Will My Hair Grow Back?

If you received chemotherapy that caused hair loss (alopecia), you can expect your hair to start growing back within weeks of your last treatment. Many people note hair growth even during their chemotherapy.

If you received radiation to your scalp, it may take weeks or months before you see some growth. How long it takes to grow and how well it grows will depend on the dose of radiation you received. High-dose radiation can cause permanent hair loss in the area of the scalp radiated.

What Will My Hair Look Like When It Grows Back?

The texture, color, and/or curl pattern of your hair may be different from what they were prior to cancer treatment. Many people are elated—when gray is gone, say, or hair is thicker, wavier, and softer. Unfortunately, some people are disappointed—when blond hair returns a mousy brown or naturally wavy hair returns frizzy and unmanageable.

The hair that first grows back may not remain the same over the subsequent months and years. For example, hair that first grows in soft may become coarser with time.

AFTEREFFECTS INVOLVING THE LUNGS

What If I Get Short-winded Easily?

A sense of being short-winded can be caused by

- direct changes in your airway or lungs from surgery, radiation, or chemotherapy
- changes in your heart
- anemia
- deconditioning (loss of tone and strength because of lack of exercise)

What If I Cough a Lot?

Coughing can be due to one of many different problems. After cancer therapy, a cough is often caused by

- effects of your cancer on your lungs or throat
- effects of your treatment on your lungs or throat
- allergies
- reflux of stomach contents into lungs
- infection

Let your oncologist know if you have a cough. If your oncologist is aware of your cough, let your oncologist know if

- your cough gets worse
- your cough prevents sleep
- your cough becomes so productive that you bring up sputum or blood
- you develop fever, chills, or shortness of breath
- you develop chest pain

AFTEREFFECTS INVOLVING THE HEAD AND NECK

What If My Eyes, Nose, and Mouth Are Dry?

Dryness can be due to

- radiation- or chemo-induced changes in the glands that supply moisture to these areas

• medication effect
• an immune disorder that damages or destroys the glands that supply moisture to these areas

What If It Is Hard to Swallow?

Difficulty in swallowing after cancer treatment can be due to

• dry mouth
• injury to the nervous control of swallowing
• radiation changes to the mouth, throat, and/or esophagus
• infection in the esophagus

Short-term radiation changes will usually resolve within a few weeks to months of completing therapy. Permanent scarring of the esophagus can occur months to years following radiation to the chest (mediastinum). This delayed scarring can cause narrowing, called stricture, of the esophagus, which is treated with dilations by a gastroenterologist (a doctor specializing in diseases of digestion).

Infections (viral, fungal) are usually quite painful and require treatment aimed at eradicating the infection.

Can Cancer Treatment Cause Cataracts?

Cataracts are common in otherwise healthy people over sixty-five years old. They can occur earlier and more frequently following

• radiation to the eye
• long-term exposure to steroids (corticosteroids, or cortisone-type drugs, such as prednisone)

Why Does Food Sometimes Taste Different after Cancer Treatment?

Treatment of head and neck cancers can result in temporary or permanent alteration in taste due to

- changes in the tongue
- diminished or absent smell sensation
- diminished saliva
- effect of medication

What Is Osteoradionecrosis of the Jaw?

This is a serious complication of radiation to the jaw and is due to bone infection. High-dose radiation to the jaw causes permanent changes that render the bone unable to respond normally to infection in the gums or teeth. This problem has become uncommon as techniques of delivering radiation have improved and attention has been given to proper care of teeth. You can prevent this complication by

- getting frequent (every three to four months) high-quality dental care
- brushing properly and flossing regularly
- seeing your dentist at the first sign of swelling of the gums or the first hint of pain in your gums or a tooth

What Are Radiation Caries?

This is an aggressive form of dental caries (cavities in the teeth) that occurs after radiation to the head and neck. Because it is usually painless, it can, if not picked up by frequent dental exams, progress to such a point that the teeth cannot be salvaged. It is caused by changes in the quality of the saliva, as well as by decreased quantities of saliva.

How Can I Prevent Radiation Caries?

You can help prevent radiation caries by

- having frequent dental exams
- practicing meticulous oral hygiene (brushing and flossing)
- applying topical fluoride every day
- eating a healthy diet

3

Practical Issues

Surviving cancer is not just about being alive. It is about quality of life. How you deal with day-to-day practical issues has a major impact on your quality of life after cancer treatment. You have to adjust to your new role as a patient in follow-up; your relation to your health care team is different from what it was when you were under active treatment. You must learn to understand how your body has changed so that you can integrate your cancer-related needs with routine medical needs having nothing to do with cancer. Vacation plans take on new twists as you consider physical and scheduling constraints. Taking medications, even over-the-counter remedies, may require more discretion and supervision. Old issues, such as a healthy diet and regular exercise, take on new urgency or pose new obstacles. Changed priorities may spur you to modify how you manage your time or your money. Changed circumstances may force you to manage old problems in new ways.

The fact that you have changed or that old habits no longer work is not terrible. Adjusting to the changes will make some aspects of your life better than they were before your cancer. Other adjustments will not make your life better, or even as good, but will make it as comfortable as possible under the circumstances.

Still other adaptations will leave your situation neither better nor worse, just different.

If you accept a wonderful new job that takes you from your home in a neighborly suburb to an impersonal high-rise in a city, you will encounter many changes. Negotiating mass transit for the first time in your life means learning the most economical and efficient routes, and adjusting to traveling at restricted times with limited baggage (no car in which to pile things you might need). No longer part of a friendly neighborhood where everyone helps everyone else, you may have to seek friendships and companionship outside your condo. You have to find a new place to shop for clothes, buy groceries, and do your laundry. An increased cost of living may force a change in money management. Although your new job may be an excellent move professionally, the accompanying changes may be good or bad, hard or easy, depending on how you deal with them.

Finishing treatment has many similarities to starting a new job. The surviving of cancer causes changes in you and your circumstances. You can choose how you respond to the differences. One response is to recognize them but to try to make your old ways work in your new life. Wanting the comfort of familiarity, you try to push the round peg of your old ways in the square hole of your new life. The roundness feels reassuring at first, but with time you feel discomfort as the misfit causes frustration and failure. Another response to the changes is to ignore or lament them, but this will not help you adjust to your new life. Or you can embrace the changes that will impel you to make life-enhancing changes and recognize the unwanted changes as a practical challenge in your new life.

The goal of this chapter is to help you adjust to the changes introduced by your cancer experience: working with your health care team, reintegrating yourself into the work and social worlds, addressing your children's needs, and establishing and developing a system of keeping up with cancer developments that affect you.

STAYING IN THE MEDICAL SYSTEM

If I Was Treated by an Oncologist, Do I Still Need an Oncologist after Completion of My Treatments?

At least for a while, you need an oncologist to

- oversee your reevaluation
- advise you regarding the appropriateness of stopping treatment
- advise you regarding follow-up (which tests and procedures need to be done when, where, and how)
- advise you regarding measures to prevent recurrent or new cancer or other medical problems.
- evaluate and treat any cancer-related and treatment-related complications, aftereffects, or side effects
- evaluate and treat early any future problems that may indicate recurrent problems with your cancer.

Will I Need to Be Followed by an Oncologist for the Rest of My Life?

Depending on your type of cancer and your personal cancer situation, after completion of cancer treatments you may need to be followed by your oncologist for a few more visits, a few more months, a few years, or the rest of your life.

If your oncologist advises that you no longer need to follow up with him or her, you are "dismissed." This means that you now can do without the expertise of a cancer specialist involved in your routine care. Under these circumstances, your oncologist feels that follow-up with your internist or family practitioner will be just as good. Since you have to see him or her anyway for routine care unrelated to your history of cancer, it will be more convenient for you to see one doctor instead of two. Even if you are dismissed, your oncologist will keep your medical file and be available for questions, problems, or reevaluations at your request or if the need arises.

If you are involved in a clinical trial, you may need to proceed with follow-up with your oncologist for the rest of your life for the sake of monitoring and data collection. This follow-up will be nothing more than an inconvenience.

Can I Switch Oncologists Now?

You can switch doctors at any time. If you feel the need to switch oncologists, now is a good time because

- your treatment is complete
- you need to be reevaluated anyway
- you are about to start a new phase of cancer follow-up

Why Would I Switch Oncologists Now?

There are a number of common reasons why you might feel the need to switch oncologists after completing your cancer treatments:

- Your oncologist is very far from your home.
- Your oncologist does not participate in your insurance plan, and your insurance will not cover your current oncologist's bills.
- You were not comfortable, confident, or satisfied with your oncologist, despite sincere attempts to make it work during treatment. You can be going to the most famous, well-respected oncologist in the world for your type of cancer. If his or her style or personality makes it difficult for you to communicate your needs, then this oncologist is not the best person to be caring for you.
- You feel that your oncologist is not interested in your care now that your treatment is complete.

Can I Continue My Routine Non-Cancer-Related Medical Care with My Oncologist?

In general, it is best to continue your routine non-cancer-related care with your internist or family practitioner, not your oncologist. Some of the reasons for this are that

- oncologists' offices are set up to diagnose and address cancer-related problems, not general medical problems
- oncology offices are not set up for routine comprehensive medical evaluations
- it is not cost-effective for you
- if a new medical problem were diagnosed, you would probably be referred to a general internist or a family practitioner

If you do not have an internist or family practitioner, ask your oncologist for a referral. If you want your oncologist to be your only doctor, discuss with him or her whether this is an option for you and whether it is in your best interests.

Which Oncologist Do I See If I Move to Another City?

In our mobile society, where it is common to move to another city, you can

- establish yourself with a new oncologist in your new hometown and have all of your cancer-related care attended to locally (your original oncologist can be kept informed of your progress and provide input on your care through telephone calls, letters, and reports)
- return to your original oncologist for routine follow-ups or if you develop a new cancer-related problem (this is not practical if you have ongoing problems or require frequent follow-up)
- continue your major checkups with your original oncologist and establish yourself with a new oncologist in your hometown who can do the brief checkups and attend to minor problems (your original and your new oncologist must both be agreeable to this arrangement)

The best choice for you will depend on

- your type of cancer
- the complexity or unusualness of your situation
- the sophistication of the local facilities

• financial concerns
• the location of family and support people

Why Do I Need to Tell All My Doctors about My Cancer History?

If you see or speak to doctors who are not oncologists, such as your gynecologist or cardiologist, be sure to tell them that you recently completed cancer therapy. Your history of cancer treatment is an important piece of information when a doctor is determining the cause of your problem and how serious the problem is or could become.

Can I Assume That Any Noncancer Medical Conditions Will Be Detected or Followed at My Cancer Checkups?

Not necessarily. Your cancer doctor tailors your evaluations to look for cancer- and treatment-related problems. Their offices and practices are not set up to perform routine comprehensive medical evaluations, such as the prevention, evaluation, and treatment of heart disease, diabetes, low thyroid, and other common medical conditions.

In fact, most oncology offices expect you to pursue your routine cancer screening for other cancers with your general medical doctor. For example, if you were treated for lung cancer, you should have your routine colon cancer screening done with your general medical doctor and your routine cervical cancer screening done with your gynecologist or general medical doctor.

Since I Have Had One Type of Cancer Already, Do I Need to Be Screened Any Differently for Other Diseases or Cancers Than Someone Who Has Never Had Cancer?

Some cancers are associated with an increased risk of another cancer. Some cancer treatments are associated with an increased risk of developing certain cancers or other medical problems. These factors will be taken into account when your routine screening regimen is planned. (See Chapter 2.)

If My Oncologist Dismissed Me, How Can I Be Sure My General Doctor Knows How to Take Care of Me Now That I Have Had Cancer?

Taking care of patients with a history of cancer is routine for internists and general practitioners. If you have any concerns about your follow-up,

- arrange for a visit with your oncologist to review the specifics regarding your follow-up
- request that your oncologist communicate with your general doctor by phone and/or letter, outlining the recommendations
- learn about the follow-up of your type of cancer from books, journals, and information hotlines, and discuss your findings with your general doctor.

Even if you are not actively followed by your oncologist, your oncologist is available for telephone or in-office consultation regarding questions, concerns, or new problems that arise at any time after completion of your cancer treatments.

Do I Need a Dental Exam?

If you received radiation that affected your mouth or if you received certain chemotherapy regimens, you need to pay extra attention to the care of your teeth and gums. It is best to have an exam before your cancer treatments in order to find and treat any dental problems. After completing your cancer treatments, it is important to have another thorough dental evaluation and an exam every three to four months for a few years. This is because you are at increased risk of tooth decay, which can be prevented with good daily hygiene and frequent professional evaluation and treatment.

If you received radiation to your jawbone, you have extra reason to be meticulous about the care of your teeth. Extracting teeth because of decay or infection increases the risk of a serious complication called osteoradionecrosis. (See the section on the head and neck in Chapter 2.)

When Do I Resume My Routine Non-Cancer-Related Medical Care?

Set up an appointment to see your general doctor in the month or two after the end of your cancer treatment. This allows your doctor to be familiar with all the changes that have taken place and with your new baseline. Your doctor can focus on all the non-cancer-related health issues.

Can I Wait a While before Getting Involved with More Doctors and, Possibly, More Tests?

After cancer treatment is completed, people tend to be weary of the expense, inconvenience, anxiety, and discomforts of checkups. However, in general, the sooner you go, the better. It is important that any new noncancerous conditions be diagnosed and evaluated, in order to

- prevent complications from the problem
- promote healing and recovery from your cancer
- help you feel better
- prevent symptoms or problems that can make you or your doctor worry about your cancer when, in fact, the symptoms or problems are due to a new, noncancerous condition.

One middle-aged woman, while recovering uneventfully from treatment for a muscle tumor, went for her routine annual mammogram. She was found to have a tiny breast cancer. At first she was overwhelmed. After getting through the shock and anger, she was glad that she had proceeded with her mammogram. The breast cancer was there whether she screened for it or not. By getting her mammogram as scheduled, it was diagnosed while small enough to be cured without chemotherapy. Delaying the mammogram, and thus her diagnosis, would have made her recovery from the muscle tumor easier but have threatened her overall health and her life. A six-month wait might have given it time to spread to the lymph nodes, thus requiring chemotherapy for any chance of cure.

An elderly man who was recovering from treatment for melanoma was reluctant to have his colon checked for cancer. He did not have any increased risk of colon cancer and was symptom-free, but he was feeling particularly vulnerable. Proceeding with his colon evaluation and getting a good report was the best medicine in the world for him.

Whom Do I Call If I Develop a Problem That May Be Related to My Cancer or Cancer Treatments?

If you are still seeing your oncologist regularly, call your oncologist. If you have been released from the care of your oncologist, call your regular physician and explain your problem. Your doctor can advise you whom to see.

Whom Do I Call If I Develop a Problem Unrelated to My Cancer, Such as Bronchitis or Backache?

Call your regular doctor, not your oncologist. If your regular doctor feels your problem may be related to your cancer or cancer treatment, he or she will consult with your oncologist or refer you back to your oncologist.

Use the medical system effectively for routine care, non-cancer-related care, and cancer-related care.

Since I Have Had Cancer Treatment, Am I at Increased Risk for AIDS?

No. Cancer and cancer treatment do not increase your risk of getting AIDS. If you received blood products, there is an extremely small risk of transfusion-associated infection.

Am I Now More Susceptible to Infection Than I Was before My Cancer?

Radiation therapy and chemotherapy cause changes in the immune system that are quantifiable by sophisticated tests but do not show up as increased episodes of illness. Chronic stress and profound grief affect the immune system and may play a role in the frequency of infectious illness.

If it seems to you that you have more infectious-type illnesses, you may indeed have more illnesses. Or you may be getting the same number of illnesses, but you notice each episode more because

- you get sicker or feel worse with each minor illness as a result of your generally weakened condition
- you are more anxious about any illness

Whether or not you are more susceptible to infection depends on

- the type of cancer you had
- the type of therapy you had
- the type of surgery you had
- your current medicines
- your nutritional status
- your age

Ask your oncologist about

- the likelihood of your being at increased risk of viral or bacterial infections
- precautions you can take to prevent infections
- signs or symptoms of infections

Do I Need Any Vaccinations?

Vaccinations are given to help prevent specific diseases. They come in many different types. Some are routinely given to almost everyone, such as the tetanus vaccine. Others are given only to people with special medical conditions, such as the pneumonia vaccine. Still others are given to anyone with an increased risk of being exposed to the disease, such as yellow fever vaccination before travel to high-risk areas, or hepatitis vaccine before the start of work with high occupational exposure.

Discuss with your oncologist and internist whether you need any vaccinations now or in the foreseeable future and whether there are any vaccines that you should avoid. Vaccinations in adults are given when the benefit outweighs the risk, such as when there is an increased risk of getting infected or an increased risk of complications from the infection. In general, adults who are at increased risk of infections and who may benefit from certain vaccinations, such as the flu vaccine or pneumonia vaccine, include those who

- are over sixty-five years old
- have significant heart, lung, or kidney problems
- have certain cancers
- are on certain medications
- have had their spleen removed
- know that they are going to be exposed to a preventable infection

Vaccinations are given in hopes of building up your body's immunity to specific infections before you are exposed to the infection. Exposure to the infectious agent after your immunity is boosted usually results in a milder illness or none at all. Vaccination does not guarantee protection, because many factors determine whether the vaccine works in you.

Vaccines containing live virus can be dangerous in certain patients. Be sure to discuss your cancer treatment with any doctor who recommends that you receive a vaccine, and discuss any plans for vaccination with your oncologist.

Why Is the Timing of Vaccination Important?

The timing of the administration of vaccines is important for several reasons:

- Your body must be able to mount an immune response to the vaccine in order for it to be effective. If a vaccine is given too soon after cancer therapy, your body may not mount an effective response.
- It takes a few weeks after vaccination to build up immunity. If you are vaccinated just prior to exposure to the illness, your body may not have had enough time to build an effective immunity.
- The resultant immunity lasts for a specified length of time. For short-lived vaccine-induced immunity, the timing of the administration of the vaccine should be such that your peak immunity will occur at the expected time of exposure to illness. If you are vaccinated too early before exposure, your immunity may have waned and become less effective when you need it.

Do I Need a Pneumonia Shot?

The pneumonia vaccine is a safe and effective vaccine that helps build your immunity to the most common cause of pneumonia, the pneumococcus. You are a candidate for the pneumonia vaccine if you

- are sixty-five or older
- have diabetes
- have chronic lung disease
- have kidney failure
- are taking drugs that suppress your immune system
- have multiple myeloma

The Centers for Disease Control advises that people in close contact (housemates, children, other close associates) with those who need the pneumonia vaccine also get vaccinated. This will minimize the chance that a contact person will bring the infection to a person at risk.

Receiving the pneumonia vaccine does not guarantee that you will never get pneumonia. It merely offers some protection against the most common cause of pneumonia. You can still develop pneumonia from one of the many other causes of pneumonia not covered by the vaccine.

Do I Need a Flu Vaccine?

In general, it is a good idea to minimize your chance of getting sick, including catching the flu (influenza). After cancer treatment, there are additional physical and emotional benefits to preventing illness such as influenza. If you do not have a history of egg allergy or some other reason for not taking it, you should probably receive the flu vaccine. Discuss with your doctor the risks to you of influenza.

When large numbers of people receive the flu vaccine, it is effective in decreasing the overall incidence and severity of flu in the group. But many factors determine how effective the flu vaccine is for each individual. Taking the flu vaccine does not guarantee that you will not get the flu.

The flu vaccine is given every fall, around October, to persons who need it. It is also available to people who simply hope to avoid the inconvenience of the flu (workers and homemakers for whom a few days "out of commission" would be a hardship).

Flu vaccines protect for only one season. You need to be revaccinated in every year in which you wish to boost your immunity to influenza.

Do I Need a Hepatitis Vaccine?

The hepatitis vaccine is recommended to people at increased risk of exposure to hepatitis B. Transfused blood undergoes extensive sensitive testing for hepatitis B prior to approval for transfusion, so the risk of transfusion-associated hepatitis B is very low. It is an expensive, three-shot regimen, usually given over six months. An optional regimen is given over two months. This type of vaccination can be discussed if there is a reasonable concern that you will need blood products in the future. For example, if you had a type of cancer that is treated with bone marrow transplantation if it recurs, then you might consider having this vaccine given to you while you are in remission.

Can My Children Proceed with Their Routine Vaccinations?

Some of the routine vaccines that children receive are "live" vaccines, namely, weakened but alive viruses. Check with your oncologist whether and when it is safe for you to be exposed to someone who has received a live vaccine.

Who Owns My Medical Records? My Scans and X Rays?

Medical records belong to your doctor, but you have a right to a copy of the records. Your scans and X rays belong to the doctor who ordered them or the radiography center where they were taken. You have a right to a copy of your X rays, but oftentimes you will be charged a copying fee.

Is It a Good Idea to Read My Own Medical Records?

For most people the disadvantages outweigh the advantages. The main reason people want to read their records is to find out about their condition. In general, if you feel you are not getting accurate or enough information about your medical condition from your oncologist, ask him or her to discuss your case with you in greater detail. If you still feel that you are not getting answers to your satisfaction, it is time to find a doctor with whom you communicate better, and not depend on self-interpretation of your records.

The advantages of reading your own medical records include

- finding out details you missed during the discussions
- verifying your understanding of your condition

A major disadvantage of reading your own medical records is the enormous potential for misinterpretation of symbols, phrases, and medical conclusions. Once you read these things, it can be difficult for you to dismiss them from your mind even if subsequent discussion clarifies your misunderstanding. Some misunderstandings are easily corrected, and even amusing ("male, c/o SOB" is a man who is complaining of shortness of breath). Other misreadings are subtle but dangerous. Your doctor's notes may indicate that "there is no evidence of metastases at this time," which is a standard phrase to document a thorough exam. You may be left with a disquieting sense that your doctor is anticipating you developing metastases, when in fact your doctor is not.

You may read things that you really did not want or need to know and that cause you unnecessary anxiety. When evaluating a patient, doctors commonly write a list of different conditions that could be causing a symptom or problem. They may be unconcerned about most of the possibilities but include them for completeness. You, on the other hand, may be left worrying about problems you had not even thought of before.

What Is a Tumor Registry?

A tumor registry is a hospital-based person or group who collects information about patients diagnosed with, or treated for, cancer at that hospital. "Tumor registry" is also the name for the bank of information. Many hospitals have developed a separate department devoted to collecting, computerizing, and analyzing this information. Usually your oncologist or primary care physician is responsible for keeping the registry informed about

- your cancer (present or absent, stable or progressive)
- any recurrences
- the initial treatment you received for your cancer
- any cancer-directed treatment you receive each year after your original diagnosis

What Happens to the Information in the Tumor Registry?

Tumor registries allow hospitals (and doctors) to follow the course and outcome of their patients diagnosed and treated for cancer. Analysis of the data is one way to gain information about the

- incidence of the various types of cancer
- relative effectiveness of various treatment options
- relative success of one hospital's treatments compared to national standards
- outcome of patients who receive various treatments

Do I Need to Continue Learning about Cancer If I Am in Remission?

Staying informed about progress in the care of people with your type of cancer will help you. At the very least, you will better understand your follow-up. In addition, depending on how comfortable you feel with medical information, knowledge will help you participate in your own care.

Much as you may want to forget that you had cancer, it is to your advantage to think about your cancer occasionally. You may be at risk of recurrent cancer. You are at risk of developing cancer that is totally unrelated to your prior cancer (having cancer does not make you immune to other types of cancer). You may be at risk for future medical problems related to your cancer or your treatments. Learning about your cancer may enable you to decrease your risks.

Every year new information becomes available about

- the causes of cancer
- the prevention, diagnosis, treatment, and follow-up of cancer
- the prevention and treatment of aftereffects

Doing research on cancer is not for everyone. You may be someone who works best with your doctors by leaving all the decision making to them. You participate in your care by being faithful with checkups and coming in for any new problems. Trying to learn about the medical issues just causes anxiety and confusion, and does not help you. Your doctors will let you know what you need to know.

On the other hand, you may feel most comfortable learning as much as you can about your cancer. You may prefer to play a more active role in the gathering and processing of information and in the decision making. Continued learning allows you to be as involved as you desire.

Keeping up will help you discuss advances that affect you. For instance, a new screening test may become available for diagnosing a recurrence of your type of cancer. If you are knowledgeable about it, you can participate in the decision of when and how to use it.

In many circumstances your personal needs and desires are a little different from what is routinely recommended for patients in your situation. You may be very interested in participating in a clinical trial, no matter what the expense, risk, or inconvenience. Since it is impossible for your oncologist to keep up with every available trial for every type of cancer, you may want to do some research yourself.

At every visit your doctor draws conclusions and gives advice. Your doctor can arrive at his or her recommendations with as little or as much input from you as you like. Use your knowledge, be it a little or a lot, to be partners with your doctor. But remember the old adage that you cannot be your own doctor. Share your questions and information with your doctor, and let him or her come to a conclusion. You are best served if, ultimately, you trust your doctor's advice.

How Do I Keep Up with Advances Related to My Type of Cancer?

If you feel comfortable reviewing medical information, you can call the Cancer Information Service's toll-free number (1-800-4CANCER) and request copies of information about your type of cancer. Every six to twelve months call to find out whether the

PDQ (Physician Data Query) file for your type of cancer has been updated again. If it has, request a copy.

Read the science and health sections of various newspapers and magazines. However, be careful, because sometimes the reporting is inaccurate or misleading. Subscribe to newsletters or journals for cancer survivors (see Appendix III). Be sure to differentiate advertising from reporting.

At your checkups review any questions or new findings from your readings. Ask your doctor whether any new development or information related to your cancer situation has appeared since your last visit. It will be impossible for your doctor to remember what you may have reviewed at prior visits, so repeat the last "news" you had been told and then see whether anything new has developed since then.

How Do I Know Whether the Articles I Read in the Newspapers and Magazines Are Valuable for Me?

Cancer issues make good news. You will see many articles having to do with your cancer—the risks, the incidence, new treatments. Some questions to consider when reading include the following:

- Was the work done at a reputable cancer center?
- Was the work done in the test tube, with animals, or with humans? You cannot draw any conclusions about your situation on the basis of test tube or animal studies.
- Was the work double-blind placebo-controlled? In double-blind placebo-controlled studies neither the patients nor the researchers know who was getting real treatment and who was getting a placebo (a substance having no medicinal value, such as a sugar pill). These studies, in general, give more reliable results.
- Was the work subsidized by an impartial source, such as the National Cancer Institute, or by a drug company with a vested interest?
- Was the treatment being recommended by an impartial scientist or by a potentially partial party, such as a drug company?

If something looks interesting or important to you,

- share the information with your oncology nurse or doctor, and have him or her get back to you about it
- call the Cancer Information Service's toll-free number (1-800-4CANCER) for advice or more information about the news item

Newspapers and Television Make It Seem That Everything Causes Cancer. Is This True?

It is nerve wracking continually to hear about new things that may be related to cancer. Reports giving conflicting information and advice make it hard to know what to believe. Many cancers are felt to be caused, at least in part, by environmental exposures. From a practical point of view, pay more attention only to those exposures about which you can do something.

Can I Travel?

Your readiness to travel depends on

- your destination
- the length of your stay
- the mode of transportation
- your current condition
- the availability of medical care at your destination
- the timing of your follow-up tests and visits
- the need for pretravel vaccinations

People have traveled around the country even during intensive cancer treatments by advance planning with their oncologists. Arranging follow-up evaluations and treatments to be administered by willing oncologists at your destination allows you to travel without interruption in your cancer treatment or follow-up. Similarly, you can arrange for a local doctor to be available to you during your trip.

What Can I Do to Maximize My Safety and Comfort during Travel?

Plan ahead. Bring

- a written list of your medications
- a written summary of your condition (diagnoses, treatments received)
- your medications, with extra doses in case your return gets delayed
- written prescriptions, in case your medication gets lost or damaged
- over-the-counter medications that work for you

MEDICATIONS

What If I Am Still Taking Many Medicines?

After completion of cancer therapy, you may need medication to treat

- temporary side effects from your cancer
- temporary side effects from your cancer treatment
- permanent changes due to your cancer
- permanent changes due to your treatment

For example, you may need medications for treatment of

- nausea, poor appetite
- pain
- mouth ulcers
- stomach or duodenal ulcers
- infection
- malnutrition
- hormonal imbalance
- constipation or diarrhea

- cough or asthma
- dizziness
- sleep disturbance
- depression
- anxiety

How Can I Keep Track of My Medicines?

Taking your medicines properly is an important part of recovery, just as it was of treatment. If you are taking more than one medicine or are taking medicines more than once a day, you will do well to buy a "pill minder" to organize your pills. The pill minder

- serves as a daily reminder to take your pills
- serves as a daily check that you have taken your pills
- lets you know whether you are running low on your pills (if you run out of medicine as you fill your pill minder for the following week, you can get a refill without missing a dose)

You should also keep a log of *changes* in your medications. If the dose of one of your routine medicines is changed, record the date and change in dose. If you are given a course of new medication, record the dates started and stopped, as well as the drug name, dose, and frequency of administration.

Details about your use of medicines are very important for evaluations of your condition and for decisions about further tests or treatments (see Appendix V).

What If I Am Reluctant to Take Prescribed Medication?

It is common for people who have finished cancer treatment to be reluctant to take any more medications. You may find yourself declining your doctor's offered prescriptions for the control of symptoms: you would rather deal with symptoms than take any more medications. Or you may forget to take your medicines even though you never forgot during your cancer treatment. After you did so much to get well, it seems inconsistent for you to turn down an opportunity for symptom control, enhanced recovery, or improved chance for durable remission. There are a number of possible explanations for this reluctance to take medicines.

Taking medicine is a crucial part of cancer therapy. It is perhaps the first time you took so many or such potent medications. If you want to create distance from your patienthood, you may avoid, consciously or subconsciously, anything that reminds you of being a cancer patient. This reluctance to take medication can work to your disadvantage, delaying your healing, prolonging side effects, allowing preventable problems to occur or progress. Instead of seeing your medicines as signs of being sick, see them as tools for speeding your recovery from patienthood.

Reluctance to take medication is often one aspect of the bigger issue of control. During cancer treatment you had little or no control over the type, timing, dosing, or administration of your medications, let alone whether you could skip a dose. After cancer treatment you can regain a sense of control by refusing medication or forgetting to take doses. You can afford to refuse or forget because it is not life threatening. This way of achieving a sense of control is often self-defeating. The little control you gain in determining what medications you take is offset by the loss of control of your symptoms or by a possible delay in your recuperation. It may help to see your choosing to take offered prescriptions as an act of control over your recovery.

See taking medicines as one way to regain control over your health.

It is also common to fear the short- or long-term effects of medications and treatments. These fears and anxieties must be suppressed during treatment for active cancer, in order to get through the treatment. After cancer treatment any additional medicine may be seen as just too much for your body and may trigger undue anxiety related to overall anxiety about the toxicity of your prior treatments. Discuss with your doctor or nurse the risks of your medications. Knowledge will help you put the risks in perspective and make a wise decision, balancing risks and benefits.

NUTRITION AND DIET

Should I Be on a Special Diet?

Your diet is an important part of recovery from cancer and should be chosen with care. The healing process continues for weeks to months after treatment is completed. Your diet provides the resources your body needs to promote healing. When your body is repairing damaged tissues and clearing toxic substances, there is an increased requirement for

- fluids
- protein
- calories

Sometimes additional dietary specifications are required to deal with

- constipation or diarrhea
- malabsorption
- allergies
- drug interactions with dietary substances
- diabetes
- heart or kidney problems

If I Was on a Low-Cholesterol Diet before I Was Diagnosed with Cancer, Should I Resume It?

After cancer treatment is completed, the top priority in choosing your diet is selecting foods that will promote recovery from your cancer and the cancer treatment.

Fat-restricted diets have a long-term goal of decreasing the risk of hardening of the arteries in people at risk. Before you are concerned about long-term goals, you need to focus on the immediate task of recovery. Letting your cholesterol be too high for a few months will have less impact on your overall health and your life than not getting adequate nutrition for healing after cancer treatment.

If you were on a low-cholesterol diet before your cancer, have your cholesterol profile rechecked. If your doctor feels that your test results indicate that you still need to modify your intake of fat, this can be done as long as your weight is not too low and your diet provides adequate fat-soluble vitamins.

Is Low Cholesterol Associated with an Increased Risk of Cancer?

Some studies suggest that extremely low blood levels of cholesterol are associated with an increased risk of certain cancers. This is preliminary information. It may be a statistical association with no cause-and-effect relationship. Or it may be that the cancer causes the extremely low cholesterol.

If you have low cholesterol, do not try to raise it in hopes of decreasing your cancer risk. There are no data to indicate that raising your cholesterol has a beneficial effect on cancer risk.

If you have high cholesterol, the long-term benefits to your health of lowering it to a normal level outweigh any potential risks.

Is a High-Fat Diet a Risk Factor for Cancer?

Some epidemiological studies indicate an association between a high-fat diet and cancers of the breast, colon, pancreas, prostate, and uterus. This does not necessarily mean that a high-fat diet causes these cancers. Studies are under way to explain the cause of the association.

What If I Lost Weight during My Cancer Treatment?

People lose weight during cancer treatment because of

- poor eating (which has many causes, both physical and emotional)

• increased calorie requirements
• poor absorption and poor utilization of calories

What Should I Do If I Lost Weight during Therapy?

Discuss with your doctor your goal weight and how you should achieve it. You will want to supplement your diet with foods of high nutritional value, not with high-calorie "junk food."

What If I Gained Weight during Therapy?

It is very common for people to gain weight during cancer therapy. This can be due to

• medications such as prednisone
• decreased activity
• fluid retention
• increased appetite because of medications or emotional stress

Some of these factors continue to affect weight even after completion of cancer therapy.

If I Am Heavier Now, How Long Will It Take Me to Lose the Weight I Gained during My Cancer Therapy?

Depending on how much weight you gained during treatment and how you are doing now, it can take three to twelve months to get back to your usual weight. You can encourage healthy weight loss by

• eating well-balanced, nutritious meals and snacks
• avoiding nonnutritious, "empty" calories
• exercising with proper supervision

Is Obesity a Risk Factor for Cancer?

Obesity is associated with increased risk of certain types of cancer, such as breast and uterine cancer. The distribution of fat may make a difference for certain types of cancer. Human studies suggest that the risk for these types of cancers is reduced if people who are overweight lose weight.

If I Was on a Special Diet Other Than a Low-Cholesterol Diet before My Cancer Treatment, Should I Resume It?

If you had some condition that required dietary modifications before your cancer, such as diabetes, hypoglycemia, or lactose intolerance, have your doctor reassess whether you still have this condition. Your doctor can advise you if and when you should resume the dietary modifications.

Your cancer or cancer treatment may have caused a change in your previous condition such that your special diet must be adjusted. Some people may no longer require dietary restrictions or modifications, whereas others may require greater restrictions.

Can I Develop a Condition That Requires Dietary Changes?

When people go for a routine complete medical checkup, the doctor checks for diabetes, high cholesterol, and other medical conditions that improve with dietary modification. Whether you have been treated for cancer or not, you still need to be checked for these conditions. Cancer does not protect you from these other conditions.

Some people discover diabetes or other conditions during or soon after cancer treatment. In many cases it is coincidence. In others the cancer or its treatment did play a role in bringing on the condition.

Can Diet Prevent Cancer?

Most cancer survivors find themselves inundated with information about cancer prevention diets. Newspapers, magazines, newsletters, television, books, and word of mouth are sources of advice about cancer prevention diets.

There are no placebo-controlled double-blind studies evaluating the effect of diet on the development of cancer or the treatment of cancer. However, there is strong statistical evidence based on epidemiological studies that diet is related to the development of certain types of cancer, so it seems likely that diet can help prevent certain cancers.

Is There a Reliable Cancer Prevention Diet?

The key to prevention is moderation and variety. Eating any food in moderation and eating a variety of foods probably afford your best protection against cancer. On the basis of current knowledge about the role of antioxidants, obesity, and nitrites in the genesis of cancer, the American Cancer Society currently offers the following recommendations for a cancer prevention diet:

- Avoid obesity.
- Eat a low-fat diet.
- Eat cruciferous vegetables (cabbage, broccoli, brussels sprouts, cauliflower).
- Avoid excessive alcohol consumption.
- Be moderate in your consumption of salt-cured, smoked, or nitrite-cured foods.
- Eat four to six helpings of fruits and vegetables daily.

What about the Stories of People with Terminal Cancer Being Cured with a Macrobiotic or Other Unconventional Diet?

Most people with terminal cancer who follow a macrobiotic (grain and vegetable) or other unconventional diet are *not* cured of their cancer by the diet. There are well-documented stories of people with "terminal" cancers being cured after following a special diet. These people failed conventional cancer therapy or declined conventional therapy, so their cure was attributed to their diet. Testimonials are inspiring but are not scientific evidence.

For these exceptional individuals, diets may have been a factor, if not the main reason, for the remarkable recovery. However, most people with the same medical condition who follow the same diet as the exceptional survivors do not respond as well. Macrobiotic and other special diets have not been shown to treat or prevent cancer dependably. The effect of these diets has never been studied in double-blind research protocols that would allow you to draw reliable conclusions about the value of these diets in treating cancer. Further research is needed to determine the safety and role of unconventional diets in the prevention of cancer.

What Are the Risks of a Macrobiotic or Other Unusual Diet?

You may have special nutritional needs while you are recovering that would not be met by a macrobiotic or other restrictive diet.

It takes a good understanding of nutrition to get a well-balanced diet when eating macrobiotically. You risk protein inadequacy if you do not eat protein-containing foods in proper combinations. You also risk vitamin deficiencies.

If you wish to pursue a special diet, be sure to let your doctor know. Review the specifics of your diet with the doctor.

Why Should I Tell My Oncologist If I Want to Follow an Unconventional Diet?

If you are embarrassed, tell your doctors you are embarrassed, but still inform them of your dietary habits. The more your doctors know about you, the better the care you will receive. Omitting information about your diet deprives your doctors of a piece of information that may affect your evaluation and treatment.

What If I Am Embarrassed to Tell My Doctors That I Follow an Unconventional Diet?

Many people fear scorn or rejection by their doctors if they choose to follow unconventional diets or treatments. Discussing your diet with your doctors will allow them to

- reassure you that your diet is sound and acceptable, or
- give you solid reasons why your diet is a problem for you now,

but probably acceptable after you are completely recovered from your treatments, or
- give you solid reasons why your diet is not the best diet for you under any circumstances, and / or
- adjust your other medications, if necessary

Doctors know that patients consider and try unconventional methods. Sharing this information with your doctors will maximize the safety of your diet. If your doctors disapprove of your dietary habits, they will still be able to take better care of you if they are aware of those habits. It is very unlikely that you would have to leave the care of your oncologist because of disagreement over your diet.

EXERCISE

What Are the Benefits of Exercise While Recovering from Cancer Treatment?

There are many potential benefits to exercising. Exercise

- increases how much you can do (your functional capacity)
- minimizes or prevents disabilities associated with treatment and with being out of condition
- preserves muscle mass, strength, and endurance
- improves circulation
- possibly enhances the immune system
- improves your appetite
- enhances your sense of well-being
- helps reduce stress
- relieves tension and anger
- releases endorphins; which are your body's natural pain killers and antidepressants
- helps restore your sense of control
- improves your self-esteem and self-image

What Kind of Exercise Should I Do?

Your choice of exercise will depend on your level of fitness, any physical limitations, the available facilities, and your preference. Walking, stationary cycling, and swimming are especially good if you are beginning an exercise program.

A basic exercise program should include

- a warm-up period with stretching exercises and light aerobics
- aerobic exercise such as walking, cycling, stair stepping, or swimming
- strengthening exercises such as weight lifting using resistance equipment
- a cool-down period

Are There Any Risks to Exercising?

You must be cleared for an exercise program and advised regarding its specifics, in order to prevent

- bleeding complications if your blood counts are too low
- injury to muscle, bone, or ligaments if you are not ready for certain exercises or not supervised in their proper execution
- heart problems, such as heart attack or heart failure
- lung problems

In general,

- you should start off slow and easy, building up gradually
- you should not be very winded, stiff, or exhausted following your exercise program
- you should check with your doctor before continuing an exercise program if you have a new pain, a new symptom, or an aggravation of a preexisting symptom or problem
- if you have been sick, such as with a cold, flu, diarrhea, or other temporary illness, wait until you have felt well for two days before resuming exercise
- do not exercise if you have a fever

Will Exercise Interfere with My Checkups?

Exercise can cause some changes in your blood test results that will be misleading. Do not do any vigorous exercise during the hours prior to blood work.

Do I Need to Participate in a Special Exercise Program?

All exercise during recovery should be supervised at least to the degree that

• your doctor is aware of exactly what exercise you are doing
• your doctor is following your progress and is aware of any symptoms or problems experienced during or after exercise

Depending on your general medical condition and the specifics of your cancer and its treatment, your doctor may

• clear you to proceed with exercise on your own
• recommend a closely supervised rehabilitation program, preferably one geared to the cancer patient

Rehabilitation exercise programs geared to heart, lung, or arthritis patients may provide the optimal supervision for your particular situation. Find out about available programs by calling your local hospitals and rehabilitation centers.

Does Exercise Affect How Well My Immune System Functions?

Studies in humans suggest that regular exercise is associated with a decrease in the number and the severity of infections in elderly people. Laboratory studies support the idea that exercise "boosts" the immune system. We need further studies to determine how this applies to healthy young and middle-aged people and to people with cancer.

A healthy immune system helps prevent infections or decrease their severity. Avoiding infections during recovery from cancer treatment would be expected to speed your overall recovery.

The immune system plays a role in how the body deals with some cancer cells. The exact role differs for different kinds of cancer. There is reason to believe that a well-functioning immune system may help some people to

- prevent cancer
- prevent a recurrence of cancer
- slow the progression of cancer
- improve the response to cancer therapy

Beware of unsubstantiated claims for methods to boost your immune system.

INSURANCE

Can I Do Anything about Rejected Claims?

Do not accept an initial rejection as the final word. If you feel a claim has been unfairly rejected

- resubmit the claim
- request an explanation for the rejection
- have your doctor's office write a letter to the insurance company validating the medical indication for the treatment

Can I Be Dropped from My Insurance?

As of spring 1994, the answer is still yes. The major changes expected in our national health care processes will, it is hoped, revise the answer in the near future. Meanwhile, if you are threatened with loss of insurance, consult experts who can provide information and advice.

Where Can I Turn for Help If I Am Having Trouble Getting Insurance?

A number of organizations provide information and assistance:

- The National Coalition for Cancer Survivorship (NCCS) has staff devoted to helping its members deal with insurance problems. Call 301-650-8868.
- Your local division of the American Cancer Society can provide information about your state and local laws and regulations on employment and insurance rights. It will not represent patients in any legal action.
- Your local insurance agent can advise and assist you.
- The Cancer Information Service's toll-free hotline (1-800-4CANCER) provides information
- Your state commission on human rights and your state rehabilitation commission provide information and assistance.
- The Health Insurance Association of America publishes a pamphlet, *What You Should Know about Health Insurance,* which you can obtain by writing to the Health Insurance Association of America, 1850 K Street NW, Washington, DC 20006.

What Is "Job Lock"?

Job lock is a predicament that arises when you feel you cannot leave your current job without risking losing your insurance coverage. This also applies to spouses, when your spouse is "locked in" to a job if you are covered under your spouse's insurance. In cases where divorce is desired, the potential loss of insurance accompanying divorce can cause "marriage lock," partners staying together solely because of insurance needs.

Do I Have to Tell Insurance Companies That I Have Been Treated for Cancer?

You cannot expect to get away with lying if there is any place on a form that asks whether you have ever had cancer or ever been treated for cancer. It is too easy for an insurance company to find out. If its investigators find out that you lied, you can be dropped from their program and be made responsible for reimbursing the insurance company for all past payments.

If the company does not ask about your past medical history or about a history of cancer, you are not obligated to volunteer it.

What Do I Do If My Company Changes the Network of Doctors and Hospitals It Will Cover, and My Oncologist Is No Longer Covered under My Company's Plan?

This is a common situation. You have established a wonderful working relationship with your doctor, you have been through rough times together, you know how to communicate with each other, and your doctor has earned your complete trust. Suddenly you find yourself faced with the decision of staying with your doctor, and paying the doctor bills out of your pocket, or switching to a new doctor.

What you decide to do depends on your circumstances. Find out from your company or your doctor whether you can be covered for at least a portion of the fees, or whether your doctor provides any unique service to you that would qualify for coverage under your plan, such as a special expertise. Inquire whether your plan intends to include your doctor again in the near future or whether you can influence your company or your doctor to stay in the plan (voiced intentions are not commitments).

If you most likely will have to pay doctor bills out-of-pocket, calculate the cost to you on the basis of the development of medical problems. The cost for routine follow-up when everything is going well may be manageable, but if you develop medical problems or land in the hospital, doctor bills can mount in a hurry. Accounting for this possibility will help you avoid having to look for a new doctor after illness strikes or to incur great debt.

A good solution is to establish yourself with a reputable doctor, possibly one recommended by your current doctor, who is covered by your plan. See this not as losing your preferred doctor but as gaining another. You and your new doctor can keep your prior doctor up-to-date regarding your progress. If problems arise, you can see your prior doctor in consultation or choose to have him or her resume your primary care. This approach relieves your worries and keeps your options open.

If your insurance plan does not cover your doctor's services, balance the value of your comfort and confidence in your current doctor against the hardship of the bills.

How Will All the Upcoming Health Care Reform Affect My Insurance?

Health care in the United States is in the process of major upheaval and change. No one can predict exactly how these reforms will affect individuals. In your own interest, let your elected officials know of your concerns and circumstances. Above all, remain informed.

MONEY

What If Money Is a Difficult Topic to Think about and Discuss?

Cancer treatment is expensive. For most people, cancer treatment strains financial resources and security because of

- the cost of the treatments
- the cost of the follow-ups
- the cost of extra help required
- the cost of accessories (wig, hospital bed, new clothes, or walking aids to accommodate physical changes)
- the lost income of the cancer survivor
- the lost income of the support person who may have taken time off to help

Cancer survivors worry about money because they worry about

- their future medical expenses
- paying their current outstanding bills (this may be the first time that they have expenses greater than their means)
- future family financial security

- difficulty in getting or keeping a job
- future financial needs from crises not related to cancer

Cancer survivors feel guilty about money because

- their cancer consumed financial resources and makes future resources uncertain
- they are often unable to contribute to the financial recovery for a while
- the topic of money, often taboo under normal circumstances, can be especially so under the strained circumstances of recovery
- they may sense resentment by others at the hardship
- people feel they are supposed to be "above" worrying about money when health is at stake

What If I Am Feeling Guilty and Worried about Money?

Find out which of your concerns are real and which imaginary. Share your concerns and feelings about your money situation with your family. Shared feelings are always more manageable. You may find out that some of your concerns were unfounded, that you are in better financial shape than you thought, or that your family truly does not resent or worry about your expenses.

If the subject of money has created genuine tensions in your family, they need to be addressed. Share your thoughts and concerns with support people and counselors if need be. Figuring out the sources of the tensions and finding workable solutions to practical and emotional issues will minimize the added strain of worry over finances.

Find out what you can do to ease your financial burdens. Get advice from financial counselors, social workers, and support groups, such as the American Cancer Society and the National Coalition for Cancer Survivorship.

Deal with your present financial concerns, and let go of distant future financial concerns for now. If you have young children at home, the year after completion of cancer treatment is not the time to worry about their college education.

WORK AND SCHOOL

What Is the Americans with Disabilities Act?

In July 1990 the Americans with Disabilities Act (ADA), providing civil rights protection to people with disabilities, was signed into law by President Bush. It guarantees equal opportunity for employment and for state and local government services, as well as equal access to public accommodations, transportation, and telephone relay services.

In July 1992 Title I became effective, banning discrimination by employers of twenty-five or more employees against a qualified employee because he or she is disabled, has a history of a disability, or is regarded as being disabled. After July 26, 1994, Title I also affects employers of fifteen to twenty-four employees.

For more information, call the Americans with Disabilities Act information hotline, at 202-514-0301.

The National Coalition for Cancer Survivorship offers the pamphlet *Your Employment Rights as a Cancer Survivor*. Call 301-650-8868.

When Will I Be Ready to Return to Work or School?

If you stopped going to, or decreased your hours at, work or school during your cancer treatments, when you will be ready to return to work or school and how full a schedule you will be able to handle will depend on

- how vigorous your treatment was
- how well you are doing physically
- how well you are doing emotionally
- how well things are going at home
- how much flexibility in scheduling your job allows

- the physical and emotional demands of your schoolwork or job
- your financial situation

Should I Return to My Old Job?

Your prior job may no longer be the right job for you, because

- physically or emotionally, you are no longer able to perform the expected duties
- you were unhappy at your job before and feel that this is a good opportunity to make a change
- you were happy at your job before, but because of the changes catalyzed by your cancer experience, you feel that it no longer provides satisfaction
- rightfully or not, you feel that your ability to function effectively has been permanently compromised because your boss and co-workers knew you during your illness

Where Do I Get Help Finding a New Job?

If you feel you must look for a new job, find out whether you qualify for a vocational training program or whether your prior employer has or knows of other job opportunities for you.

Do I Have to Tell Prospective Employers about My Cancer History?

No. Under the Americans with Disabilities Act, a prospective employer may not inquire about medical problems except as they might interfere with your ability to perform the duties required by the job. You are not obliged to undergo a medical examination until after the job has been offered.

Should I Tell a Prospective Employer about My Cancer History?

Whether or not you tell a prospective employer will depend on

- whether secondary effects of your cancer or its treatment might interfere with your job performance
- whether the type of relationship you expect to have with your boss would be hampered by withholding information about your cancer history or enhanced by sharing the information

What Are the Advantages of Telling My Boss or Co-workers about My Cancer?

Sharing your cancer history can be beneficial for many reasons. If you have some residual changes that are obvious, such as visible healing scars, the need to void very often, or a chronic cough, there will be no misunderstanding about why you look or act the way you do. You will not have to put up quite as convincing a front on difficult days. It can be stressful to try to hide the fact of your cancer history and to try to figure out how someone else might deal with it if he or she found out. You will not have to create excuses or explanations when you need to make schedule changes for tests and checkups.

Another benefit of informing your co-workers and boss about your cancer is that you may find an important support system at work.

What Are the Disadvantages of Sharing Your Diagnosis at Work?

There may be significant disadvantages to sharing your diagnosis at work. For example,

- you may have to deal with others' concerns, fears, or prejudices about your situation ("Any sign of recurrence?")
- people's genuine concern may remind you about your cancer on days when you would have forgotten about it ("How are you doing? When is your next checkup?")
- you may be disappointed by some people's discomfort with your situation, or by their lack of concern or sympathy when you need it

DEALING WITH YOUR CHILDREN

What Do I Tell My Children about My Health after My Treatment Is Completed?

What you tell your children will depend on what you have told them so far, how they are dealing with your illness, how old and mature they are, and what the specifics of your circumstances are.

In general, it is best to tell them the truth about all aspects of your health that affect them. Inform them whether you have any cancer left, whether you need any further treatments, and what to expect over the next few weeks to months (as much as you can predict). Everything should be said in a hopeful and optimistic way.

Be prepared to repeat yourself over the next few months and years. Your children will hear only what they are ready to hear. As they mature, even week to week, they become ready to absorb more information.

Do I Need to Tell Them Everything?

Absolutely not. You need to talk to them only about things that affect their world. You do not have to tell them every time you go for a checkup. However, if you have to take your children with you, or if you are going to come home with Band-Aids in your elbow creases, then they must be told. If you leave it to their imagination to figure out why you were at the doctor, they will very likely come up with a more frightening reason than your routine cancer follow-up.

You do not need to report every symptom you have. However, if you suffer headaches or irritability from your medication, or if you have pain that makes it difficult to walk long distances, tell them. Otherwise, you leave it open for your children to conclude that you are irritable because you are unhappy or angry *with them*, or that you do not want to go to the park, because you do not want to be with them. They may not be happy about your limitations, but they will understand.

Children should be protected from the anxiety of waiting for test results and from the ups and downs of evaluating potential problems. Your children do not need to know that your blood tests indicate a slight elevation of liver enzymes and that your doctor is going to recheck it in two weeks. When you know something definite that will change the circumstances at home, let your children in on it.

Try to avoid telling them about problems about which they cannot do anything. They cannot appreciate, let alone affect, your concerns about the medical bills. If your medical expenses necessitate a noticeable change in lifestyle, you can present it as a fact of life that your treatments are expensive. You would pay for treatments for any member of the family, and you are glad that the treatments are available. Feeling sorry for your children tells them to feel sorry for themselves. Adjusting to the change in financial status teaches your children about sacrifice as well as about facing challenge and loss.

What Do My Children Need?

Children require continuous satisfaction of their basic physical and emotional needs. You have to provide food and shelter, transportation to school and after-school activities, love, and comfort for their hurts.

Your children have to understand what they see going on around them, on their level. They will try to understand why you are tired or why you are still going for checkups, whether you talk about it or not.

Your children need reassurance that their needs will be met. Although their concerns may pale next to yours, fulfilling them offers great stability. Birthday parties may feel like a stressful inconvenience to you, but they are important to your children. Postponing or canceling these celebrations would disappoint them and could cause them anxiety by conveying the message that something is seriously wrong.

Remembering these three basic needs will help you prioritize your responsibilities to your children, and find the right words to comfort and reassure them:

- satisfaction of their physical and emotional needs
- a truthful explanation, appropriate to their age, of what is going on
- reassurance that their needs will be met

Do I Have to Tell Them the Truth?

It is crucial that you tell your children the truth, in order that they can trust you. The importance of this trust is amplified by the uncertainties and stress surrounding your health. Children are resilient and can handle challenge, loss, and uncertainty. They can accept your losing a body part or function, needing ongoing treatment, or living with a chance of recurrent cancer. When they see you as the same loving, caring parent despite physical changes, they are learning a powerful lesson about the value of the inner self and the triviality of appearances. Telling white lies to protect them ("My cancer cannot come back") handicaps them by making their world unreliable and untrustworthy.

Good communication with you is your children's best defense against frightening news stories or people's gossip that may give wrong information about cancer and about your condition.

If you achieve remission, you would naturally like to reassure your children that your cancer will never come back. This would seem to protect the children from worrying about recurrence, as well as to help you believe that you are going to stay well. Unless you have a 100 percent guarantee that you will not have a recurrence, you are taking a risk that can destroy the foundation of trust between you and your child. If you ever develop recurrent cancer, or your child learns that most cancers have a chance of recurrence, you will either have to continue the lie or admit to having provided erroneous information. It will be less stressful for you to help your children adjust to the truth than to maintain an untruth and worry about being exposed.

You can minimize your children's fear and anxiety about the truth by choosing how much you tell them and how you tell them. If you explain, "The cancer is gone. My doctors think that it won't come back. If it does, I'll get more treatment. There might be a new, easier way to treat it by that time, too. I'm going to plan on its not coming back, but if it does, I'll be ready to be treated again. We dealt with my cancer this time, and we can deal with it again," you offer truth, comfort, and hope in the same breath. This is the key to communication with children.

What Do I Tell the Children If My Prognosis Is Grim?

If you are doing well now, but this reprieve is expected to be short-term, or you are not doing well and the prospects for improvement are slim, you can help your children deal with this reality. It is a tragedy if your children have to deal with your terminal illness. It is a greater tragedy if you shield them from the facts of your illness. They need and deserve a chance to say good-bye and to find healthy ways to anticipate and cope with their loss. If you mislead them or deny them open communication, they will find it difficult to trust the world around them, a handicap that could follow them into adulthood.

Focus on the good things you had in the past and that you have in the present. Validate their fears, anxiety, and grief. Reassure them that their needs will be met no matter what happens to you.

What Facts Do Children Need to Know?

There are some basic facts about cancer that need emphasis. These facts will help your children deal with your illness and grow up into adults with healthy attitudes.

Make it clear that cancer is not contagious ("catchy"). Your children cannot catch cancer from you, and you cannot catch cancer from them. Make a comparison to something with which they are familiar, such as a broken leg or a headache. This point needs to be made clearly and repeatedly during and after your treatments.

Tell them the name of your cancer. By using the word "cancer," it becomes an ordinary term, and not forbidden or emotionally charged. Teach them that there are many different kinds of cancer. Breast cancer is very different from bone cancer. Even two people with the same kind of cancer can have very different illnesses. This is similar to one boy's having a little break in his leg bone and being treated with a walking cast for six weeks, and another boy's having a shattered leg bone and being treated in the hospital for six months. Both boys had broken leg bones, but their injuries were quite different. Everyone is unique.

Tell your children when changes are expected and how you will deal with them. Let them know if you expect to be tired for a few months and that you will be taking naps. Let them know when your hair will start to grow back or when you will need to have surgery. If you do not tell them, they may come to their own conclusions. They could worry that your fatigue means that you still have cancer even though the doctors said you did not. Your hair regrowth could signal recurrent cancer to them. Surgery to prevent cancer in a remaining breast (prophylactic mastectomy) or to remove an orthopedic pin could be frightening without their knowing the reason for the surgery.

Let them know that there may be unanticipated changes or problems. Reassure them that you will keep them informed and that there will be people (you, relatives, friends, and so on) to help them deal with everything.

Children notice everything. They try to understand what is going on around them and to find ways to cope. If you include them, you can guide them to accurate, healthy, and hopeful interpretations of the events. Open communication builds a deep trust that you can all enjoy from now on. Seeing your children adjust to the truth will comfort you, and may show you new ways to cope.

How Much Can My Children Handle?

Your children will tell you how much they can handle. Pay attention to their body language, comments, and questions to gauge their readiness for a topic. If they are fidgeting, avoiding eye contact, changing the topic, or trying to leave the room, they are telling you that they are not ready to talk about the topic.

Answer questions as simply and directly as possible. In general, the simpler your answers, the better. You can always elaborate if they ask for more.

Stay accessible so that information, comfort, and reassurance are provided when they most need it. Keep the other significant people in your children's lives involved. Teachers, clergy, friends' parents, coaches, grandparents, and neighbors are all in a strategic position to provide you with feedback on how your children are doing and to reinforce your communications.

Is It Okay If My Children See Me Cry?

Ideally, news and problems should be presented by you or your spouse, or both. If you are sobbing uncontrollably, your children will be afraid no matter how perfect your choice of words. Simple crying or teariness is appropriate; it teaches them that this is difficult for you and that it is normal and healthy to have and show emotions. Explain your tears: "Mommy is sad about having to go into the hospital for tests, but I'm ready to do whatever I need to do to stay healthy." "Daddy is sad about my headaches, but the doctors are going to find medicines to make them go away."

Why Am I So Impatient with My Children?

After a brush with life-threatening illness, you feel that your priorities have been clarified. Grateful for every day and all its gifts, you may regard impatience with your children as a mockery of all that you have learned about life.

There is a logical reason for your impatience. Children live in a self-centered world. Their unending demands and needs are accentuated by their impatience and short attention spans. Their coping mechanisms and priorities are immature, shaping their approach and solutions to problems. It takes energy-requiring insight and patience on your part to understand their viewpoint and respond in a mature, appropriate way.

You, as their parent, are trying to fulfill their basic physical and emotional needs while teaching them the subtleties of morality, patience, and virtue. Teaching children is a tough job under ideal circumstances.

After cancer your physical and emotional stores may be depleted. You may be dealing with your own anxieties and fears, which drain your energy in an unproductive way. You may be irritable and hypersensitive. You may just be overtired. The task of raising your children is waiting for you whether you feel ready or not.

An architect who had completed his cancer treatments was doing well except for fatigue and difficulty in concentrating. Usually soft-spoken yet strict, he found himself being slack on rule enforcement and yelling at his young children every time they whined or cried. He felt guilty that he was too tired to play with them and angry that they were making his life more difficult.

A Mercedes is a good car, but it will not run without gas and oil. This architect was a good dad who needed rest and assistance. His children needed someone who was physically and emotionally able to respond to their needs. Until the dad had the physical and emotional reserves, he had to share his fathering with other adults (friends, child care, relatives).

After resting and receiving emotional support, he was less fatigued and could concentrate better. This allowed him to be sensitive to his children's needs and respond in a helpful manner. The children were not as frustrated and whined less. He had the energy to reestablish and enforce discipline, which reassured the children.

He required naps for many months after completing his cancer treatments and participated in a support group for years. Taking the time to attend to his own needs enabled him to be a good parent and enjoy quality time with his family.

Who Can Help Me with My Children?

There are many resources for help and advice. School teachers, pediatricians, clergy, social workers, psychologists, and child psychiatrists are able to offer experience, knowledge, and energy for coping with your family's stress as a result of illness. These people can help you prevent problems with your children and pick up problems early. They can help you shoulder the children's demands for attention and their other emotional needs. And they can be there for you, the parent.

Just as you may have needed assistance with meals and carpooling during your cancer treatments, you may need some help during the months of your recovery after treatments. You may be reluctant to ask for help, because it may be less obvious to others that the need is still there. After all, you are done with treatments. Let friends and family know how they can help. During the transitional months of recovery, it is better for everyone if you use what energy you have in order to be with your children, not to make meals and do laundry.

4

—

Emotional Issues of Survivorship

THE SWORD OF DAMOCLES REVISITED: ESCAPING THE FEAR OF RECURRENCE

A tale recounted by the ancient Roman philosopher Cicero has much to teach the cancer survivor about living with fear and uncertainty. According to Cicero, Dionysius the Elder of Syracuse enjoyed enormous wealth and power, but lived in constant fear of assassination. His inability to trust anyone made him desperately lonely. One day a subject, Damocles, was praising with awe and jealousy all the wealth and luxuries enjoyed by Dionysius. Damocles declared, "All these wonderful things must certainly make you the happiest man alive." Dionysius offered Damocles the opportunity to experience royal "happiness" himself.

Damocles was made comfortable on a golden couch, near an elaborate banquet of edible delicacies. Beautiful servants attended to his every wish. Damocles was enjoying himself immensely. Dionysius then ordered that a large, gleaming sword be suspended from the ceiling by a horsehair in such a way that the tip of the blade hovered inches above Damocles' neck.

Damocles could no longer enjoy any of the surrounding luxu-

ries. Eyes fixed on the sword at his neck, he was completely para-
lyzed by his perception of the looming threat. In the end, he
begged to be released from his torturous "happiness" and allowed
to return to his normal life.

Cicero's message for us is that happiness is out of the question
if you are perpetually menaced by some terror. Damocles could
escape his terror by stepping out from under the sword. Unlike
Damocles, you will not be freed by a change of locale. As a cancer
survivor, you can escape your sword only by confronting the reali-
ties of your cancer and finding a proper place for it in your life.

What is that proper place? Can the cancer survivor ever really
escape the terror of cancer? Many people believe that survivors
must resign themselves to living forever with the fear of recurrence, illness, and death. Such resignation is not a useful or
healthy way to confront life after cancer.

The fact is that many cancers are now curable or treatable, ren-
dering the cancer survivor as healthy as someone who has never
had cancer. For these survivors, the image of the dangling sword
is simply not justified from a medical point of view. Yet too many
of these healthy cancer survivors live the rest of their lives waiting
for their recurrence. They never feel healthy, normal, or free of
their cancer, no matter how many checkups or CAT scans indicate
that they are. This feeling is often reinforced by friends and family
who view the survivor as a doomed individual and who ask, "Any
sign of a recurrence yet?" Such survivors are trapped under a
sword of Damocles, and can never be truly happy or live a normal life.

Other survivors must live with cancer or with a high likelihood
of recurrence. Yet happiness and fulfillment are still possible if
they can only tame the terror.

What you must do in order to feel normal again is step out from
under the sword and learn to perceive your life differently. Your
fear of cancer is a state of mind. You cannot choose not to have
cancer or a cancer history. But you *can* choose how you live with
your cancer or cancer history. You can learn ways to focus on your
present life and not your risk of recurrence or future illness.

You can diminish the fear, anxiety, and immobility that accompany the image of a dangling sword by mentally creating a distance so that the sword is but a dot in the landscape, or by mentally turning away so that the sword is but a vague shadow in your peripheral vision. Each of these mental exercises blunts or blocks the impact of your fear on your day-to-day experiences.

One characteristic that separates humankind from other animals is our awareness of our own mortality. We all live under its sword. Each and every one of us could end up in the emergency room on any day with an illness or injury that could become life threatening. No one is really safe. However, people who have never been seriously ill or injured generally cannot picture their end, which makes it easier for them to deny that there is one. After you have had cancer, the possible and, in many cases, probable cause of your death now has a name and a face. Being a cancer survivor, you have seen the sword up close. For you, denial of dying and death is difficult, if not impossible.

Instead of repressing fears of recurrence, future illness, or death, you can learn skills to face these fears and thus lessen or eliminate them. The risk of recurrence is a reality. The point is that no matter how great or small this risk, you can step out from under the sword by focusing on what you can do to stay healthy, prevent recurrence, and detect recurrence early.

Consider an analogy: Most of you could walk the length of a six-inch-wide beam placed on the floor. With the ground just inches away, you would focus on the beam and maintain your balance easily. If this same beam were raised five feet above the ground, most of you would weave and waver, flapping your arms as you tried to maintain your balance before falling off to the side. The beam would be exactly the same, yet the distraction of the ground five feet below would cause you to lose touch with the beam and lose your balance. Gymnasts learn to focus on the beam, not the ground. With practice, they rarely fall. When they do fall, they get right back on the beam. You, as a cancer survivor, must learn to focus on your present life, not on the uncertainties and unknowns of your future. It is a skill that can be learned and must be practiced. It will liberate you from the sword.

For all cancer survivors, especially those with an unfavorable prognosis, the cliché "quality not quantity" is very profound. By developing a frame of mind that allows you to live fully in the present, you learn a new way to measure time. By treating each day like a precious gift, you catch the moments and slow the clock of life. At worst, you fit more living into a smaller number of days. At best, you live an average number of years but squeeze many lifetimes of pleasure and experiences into them.

This chapter will help you understand and tame your terrors, as well as address other emotions, such as anxiety and loneliness, that affect your day-to-day life. It takes up such psychosocial issues as strained relationships, the resurfacing of old problems, loss of self-esteem, the role of positive thinking, and the age-old question "Why me?"

Providing a healthy framework for thinking about your feelings, relationships, and deepest fears will help you find a new normal life after cancer.

FEELINGS

How Am I Supposed to Feel As I Complete My Therapy?

The completion of therapy is usually accompanied by many different, seemingly contradictory, feelings. You may feel any combination of relief, anxiety, confusion, a sense of unreality, fear, anger, and depression. Your feelings may be mild or intense, exhilarating or frightening. They may fluctuate from day to day, even hour to hour. Take comfort in knowing that you will not always feel this way. These emotions will smooth out. Your life and emotions will seem more normal with time.

What you feel is less important than what you do with these feelings. When you have intense emotions, share them with someone you trust. Somehow, after an empathetic friend, relative, or counselor listens, you will feel better, even if you do not find any new answers. You do not move your refrigerator very often, but when you do, you would not think of moving it yourself. Completing cancer treatment is an exceptional circumstance. Why should you try to manage the emotions yourself?

If you feel like crying, find a safe place and cry until you do not feel the need any more. If you feel angry, find a safe place to vent your anger, or engage in an activity such as exercise or writing that will release some of the pent-up energy.

Try writing down your thoughts and feelings. Keeping a diary will provide a safe outlet for all your emotions and help you sort out some of your thoughts and feelings. Writing can be therapeutic, even if you throw away everything you write.

Most of your intense thoughts and feelings will fade as you move farther away from your recent experiences with cancer. If you capture them now, you will be able to remember what was happening at this time of your life. Your diary will allow you to look back and see how far you have come. Other forms of writing, such as letters and poems, provide the added dimension of being able to share with others.

There are times when the best way to handle a rough day is to go to bed early and start again tomorrow. Rest and escape are sometimes better than all the talking, analyzing, hugging, or exercising in the world. Obviously, going to bed does not change anything or solve problems. It just allows you to settle down, recharge your batteries, and start over.

What feelings you experience is less important than what you do with these feelings.

What Is the Difference between Denial and Repression?

Denial is an abnormal refusal to acknowledge the known truth. If you refuse to believe that there is any reason to have follow-up or if you deny the presence of a new lump, you are said to be in denial.

Repression is the rejection of painful or frightening ideas from conscious thought. You may have a high chance of recurrence, but you are doing well now. You are said to be repressing thoughts of recurrence if, while you are enjoying an activity, you put out of your mind thoughts about potential future problems. You know and accept all the truths, but you do not let yourself think about them all the time.

Many people use the term "denial" when they are really referring to repression.

Is Denial Healthy?

Denial is unhealthy if it keeps you from doing the right thing. Denial that prevents you from taking steps to avoid or minimize problems is harmful. If you were treated for malignant melanoma (a type of skin cancer), and you continue to spend hours in the sun with your skin unprotected, you are denying your vulnerability. Consequently, you are missing one important and easy way to help keep yourself healthy. Using sunscreen does not mean that you are vulnerable and afraid; it means that you are taking control of your situation as much as possible.

Healthy denial can bring you physical and/or emotional comfort in painful or hopeless circumstances. The story of a young woman with aggressive cancer who was deteriorating rapidly illustrates how denial can be healthy. She was bald and jaundiced (yellow from liver failure). She had done everything possible to fight her cancer and had accepted that her death was near. She shared her sadness about dying. The interesting thing was that she always acted as if she looked wonderful, referring to her pretty skin and thick hair. She knew exactly what her situation was, but her physical appearance was so abhorrent to her that her mind protected her. Her denial did not change any of her decisions. It simply shielded her from the pain of acknowledging her physical deterioration and helped her to live fully within the severe constraints of her terminal condition.

Is Repression Healthy?

Repression can be a healthy, adaptive way of dealing with a painful reality. Repression can allow you to take steps to recover or stay healthy, while minimizing the negative impact of these actions.

Fear of recurrence can be a debilitating problem, destroying your quality of life even when things are going well. Understanding and sharing this fear will diminish it, but not make it disappear completely. Repression of any remaining fear will free you to live your life most fully. Effective repression enables you to minimize your fear of recurrence between checkups, but it does not misguide you into believing you no longer need them or can ignore symptoms. Repression allows you to forget *when it is safe to forget.*

Repression is a dynamic process. When you are due for a checkup or develop a worrisome symptom, you will be less able to repress your fears. Accept the anxiety as part of a mechanism that is working well.

Repression is a healthy way of coping with physical and emotional pain as long as it does not prevent you from doing the right thing.

As you can see, repression and denial can be good or bad, adaptive or maladaptive, depending on how they are used. Repression is not inherently good or bad, any more than a drug is inherently good or bad; it depends on how it is used.

What If I Feel Relief?

After completion of cancer therapy, you may feel relief because

- your cancer was controlled
- you survived your cancer treatment
- you can retire from the full-time or part-time job of being a cancer patient
- your time and schedule will be more your own
- the emotional and physical discomforts that accompany treatment are behind you
- you will not need as much help as you did during treatment
- this chapter in your life is behind you

What If I Feel Anxious?

Many people expect all the anxiety to disappear after treatment is over. In fact, many cancer survivors actually become more anxious after treatment ends. The completing of treatment is a time for drawing conclusions and making major decisions. Is the cancer completely gone? Did I receive enough treatment? Is there anything else we can do to maintain this remission? Having choices and making decisions is anxiety producing, especially when the decisions are so important. Once these decisions are made, the anxiety will diminish.

Completing your cancer treatment and the consequent decreased contact with your health care team can be a source of anxiety. Traumatic as treatment may have been, you were reassured by knowing that while you were getting it, you were doing something active to control your cancer. Many people worry that a remaining cancer cell will multiply in the absence of treatment.

After treatment is over, you may also feel anxious about not being screened and followed as closely as you were when you were being treated. No matter how much you disliked the doctor visits and treatments, it was reassuring to have someone check you frequently. Being told to come back for a checkup in what seems like a distant three to four months can be unsettling.

In addition, as health professionals become less involved in your recovery, you may feel more responsibility for your own health and continued recuperation. Professionals and friends helped shoulder the emotional and practical burdens of your illness when you were sick. Their withdrawal after treatment can leave you feeling somewhat abandoned even though you understand rationally that their intensive involvement is no longer needed.

After treatment, at home and at work, anxiety may accompany your trying to figure out how much you can do physically and emotionally. Your reserves are depleted. You are balancing your needs for recuperation against others' seeming needs and demands. It is hard to predict the pattern or speed of your recovery, and that just adds to the anxiety.

There is the anxiety that something you do, eat, or even think may encourage the cancer to come back. You are more self-conscious about aspects of your behavior that you used to take for granted.

There is free-floating anxiety that something else may happen to you or someone you love. After all, the impossible happened once. You worry that it could happen again (see the section on Fear, page 260–71).

You may be on medication that makes you feel anxious. Your body's chemistry may have been affected by your cancer or your cancer treatment in such a way that you experience the side effect of anxiety. For example, many women undergo menopause as a result of their treatment. Anxiety can be a side effect of lack of estrogen.

Some of your anxieties related to your cancer diagnosis and treatment may be repressed during treatment. This is a common, normal adaptive mechanism for getting through the ordeal. Once the distraction of your treatments is gone, you may grasp the full impact of your situation and your experiences, and this can cause significant anxiety.

If I Am Experiencing Posttreatment Anxiety, How Long Will It Last?

Anxiety will come and go, especially around special times such as checkups and anniversaries. Recognize that anxiety is a common companion during the transition to your new normal life. The intensity and duration of your anxiety will depend on your normal tendency toward anxiety, your personal circumstances, and your reaction to your anxiety. In general, it helps when things are going well medically. The more confidence you have in your recovery and the more quickly you can return to normal activities, the less you will suffer from anxiety.

If I Am Anxious, How Can I Diminish My Anxiety?

Anxiety will not help you in any way. It wastes emotional and physical energy. Ask your doctor whether any of your medications could be causing or worsening your symptoms of anxiety. Sometimes you can alleviate anxiety by adjusting the dose or choice of your medications. You may benefit from short-term use of anxiety relievers, such as minor tranquilizers, while you pursue the other methods of anxiety reduction that take longer to be effective. It helps to avoid any stimulants, such as caffeine, or decongestants. Although your morning cup of coffee may not be causing your anxiety, it may be making the symptoms worse.

Try to determine what factors are causing anxiety. Many times it takes talking with friends, support groups, and counselors to identify what is making you anxious.

In the case of anxiety-provoking factors over which you have some control, such as worry about doing the right things to prevent recurrence or about your spouse's being impatient with the slowness of your recuperation, you can help by getting information. Knowledge will enable you to get rid of the source of your anxiety. You will relax when you know that you are doing the right things to prevent recurrence and when you are reassured that a spouse's impatience is a natural part of readjustment after cancer treatment.

In the case of anxiety-provoking factors over which you have no control, such as concern about whether you will be alive to see your grandchildren or worry about whether your car will last three more years, you can help by

- accepting that you can affect your future but that, ultimately, your future is out of your control
- training yourself not to worry about things that may not happen
- exposing concerns that are unrealistic, so that they are no longer concerns
- training yourself to not spend time worrying about things that may happen in the future but are not happening now (distract yourself from realistic worries, or repress realistic worries in a healthy way)
- being hopeful that future problems can be treated when they arise
- recognizing that anxiety is only hurting you

- praying to God, if you are a believer or want to become a believer, to attend to these things
- learning self-relaxation techniques so that you can have some control over your anxiety reactions
- getting adequate sleep (sleep deprivation can make you feel anxious, lose perspective, and think irrational thoughts)
- getting exercise, when possible
- joining a support group to share your anxieties and hear practical advice about relieving your anxieties from people who have experienced them
- talking with a survivor who is farther along the road to recovery and who is doing well
- seeking the advice and assistance of a professional counselor

Persistent anxiety drains your emotional and physical resources. Learning how to diminish and tame your anxiety will enhance your comfort and speed your recovery.

What If I Feel Emotionally Confused?

After completing treatments, people describe fluctuating emotions and thoughts. Within minutes or hours, some people shift back and forth from feeling secure to insecure, happy to unhappy, excited to listless, confident to not confident, or mellow to irritable. Changing emotions are confusing.

One man in remission felt depressed about his patch of baldness from radiation and fatigued from walking with a limp caused by a healing fracture. Then he saw a man who was terminally ill. Realizing how well he was doing overall, he suddenly felt grateful and energized.

A young newlywed felt exhilarated because for the first time since her bone marrow transplant she felt well enough to prepare a candlelight dinner for her husband. When the roast came out overcooked, she plummeted to despondency.

Another source of confusion is that you have lost the direction, structure, and focus that treatments gave your days and weeks. If you have not settled into a new routine, you are uncertain about what you should be doing. If you have ongoing medical problems, it may be a while before you can find a new routine.

Many basic questions arise after treatment that cause confusion: How healthy am I? Who is my primary caregiver? What is my role at home? How much can I do? How much should I do? How much do I want to do? What can I do? Uncertainty about these elemental questions leads to a sense of confusion.

While you were under treatment, your physical condition and the advice of your doctors and nurses helped determine your limits. Now your side effects may be less obvious and less consistent, and concrete advice about your limits may be lacking. Bewilderment arises from the need to draw limits but not knowing where or how to draw them.

You may be faced with many difficult decisions related to treatments, follow-ups, work or school, insurance, and possibly even relationships with family, friends, and co-workers. Fatigue, anxiety, and pain may make it more difficult to address these pressing issues. If you are finding it hard to prioritize, you may be trying to address many different issues at once. This leads to a clouding of the issues.

As a result of your ever-changing energy level, you may unknowingly be sending your family and friends mixed signals about whether you want extra help or can be expected to resume your old responsibilities. At the same time, their attempts to be sensitive may be sending *you* mixed signals about their concern and expectations and thereby causing you to feel puzzled.

Your medical condition may have lingering effects on your attention and memory, making it difficult for you to process all this information and responsibility. Some medicines cause confusion, as does sleep deprivation.

What Can I Do If I Feel Confused?

Things you can do to diminish your sense of confusion include

- prioritizing your responsibilities, then attending to the most important, most immediate ones

- simplifying your questions and concerns (writing them down may help you clarify them)
- getting, or having someone help you get, more information, so that you can find satisfactory answers to your questions (if your questions all end up being unanswerable or if you cannot prioritize your responsibilities, you will benefit from outside guidance in forming your questions and organizing your priorities)
- getting help from friends, family, and your health care team

Confusion is a symptom like pain, fatigue, or blurred vision. Do not be embarrassed about being confused. Let your nurse, doctor, and family know. Bringing attention to your confusion will

- minimize the risk to your health
- minimize the risk that people will misinterpret your actions
- help clarify the confusion
- avoid preventable delays in your recovery

What If Things Seem Unreal after Treatment Is Completed, As They Did When I Was First Diagnosed?

In the realm of everyday events, our subconscious is ready to accept what we experience, so we perceive our experiences as real. When events or emotions are intense or extraordinary, and our subconscious is not yet ready to integrate the information, we perceive them as unreal. They become real with time, as the subconscious develops a readiness to accept the reality.

During cancer therapy you spent weeks or months suppressing the feared outcomes, and you rehearsed in your mind life after treatment. The heightened emotions that accompany being reevaluated, coupled with end-of-treatment physical effects, can make any news seem unreal, even good news.

During treatment you spent a lot of time focused on your treatments, hospitals, and doctor visits, and in an environment such as the doctor's office where having cancer is the norm. As you spend more time in settings where most people are well (school, work, shopping malls), the apparent contrast between you and those around you will make things seem unreal. This sense is heightened by your feeling different in a place that used to be familiar. This is similar to when you visit a former home or your old school. Everything looks familiar, and yet it feels different because *you* are different.

It can take days to weeks for things to seem real again. If it is taking longer than you think it should, or the feeling is lasting longer than a few weeks, get some outside guidance.

What If I Feel Angry?

During cancer treatment you may have been too sick or too busy to appreciate certain aspects of what was happening to you. For example, you may not have cared about your inability to drive, loss of fertility, or limp, because you were focused on your fight to stay alive. Now that you have survived your treatment, you recognize the implications of the losses that you sustained earlier. These losses can make you feel angry.

You may feel angry that you "lost" time that you were hoping to use building or capping your career, raising your family, or relishing retirement. You may be angry that you were traumatized physically or emotionally by your cancer or its treatment. You may be angry that the stress of cancer has strained or crushed relationships that might have survived if not for the cancer.

In addition to old losses that you are experiencing only now, you may be experiencing new losses and problems, many of which seem unfair, such as canceled insurance, lost job opportunities, new complications from your past cancer or cancer treatment, or the need for ongoing treatments for residual noncancer medical conditions. Your cancer is gone, but now you may have a seizure disorder, heart or kidney problems, chronic cough or shortness of breath, or debilitating fatigue. More doctor visits, more tests, more expense, more uncertainty. More patienthood. You may be thinking, "Haven't I suffered enough?"

How angry each loss makes you feel is affected as much by how you see it as by what it actually is. Life is about ongoing challenges and losses, temporary or permanent, expected or unexpected, insignificant or life altering. The changes accompanying cancer are consistent with the overall rhythm of life.

As you anticipate leading a normal life again, you may be facing extra work and extra hurdles just to return to where you were before you were sick. You may expect your colleagues at school or work to be alive to your needs and provide the necessary leeway to help you ease back. Unfortunately, you may be expected to perform at least up to full force, in order to prove that you are ready to work. You may feel angry for being, in essence, punished for going through the trauma of cancer.

Lastly, you may feel disproportionate anger toward people and circumstances when things do not go well at work or at home. Since your cancer was not a person, any anger you may feel toward your cancer may end up getting directed at someone or something that also makes you angry. For example, you may feel explosive anger toward someone who turned you down for a job. It may be not that the job was so important but that you can express anger to a person but not to cancer. Besides, the person could have chosen to hire you, so you may feel anger that, with a choice available, things did not turn out well. Your cancer left no choice. Another example is anger at a loss, such as the loss of fertility. You may have had no intention or desire to have any more children, but the fact that the decision was made for you angers you.

Not only does anger come from many sources; it is often mixed with grief, anxiety, and fear. To further stir the pot, you may feel that anger make no sense if your priorities have changed. Things that you consider relatively unimportant in the grand scheme of life should not make you angry, and yet they do. You really believe that a job rejection or someone's inappropriate comment is relatively unimportant, and yet it triggers anger. It is natural that these things affect you. Even when you have settled in to your new priorities, and when job rejections or inappropriate comments bother you less, you may still have a reaction because the issues remain important in the short run.

What Should I Do If I Am Experiencing Anger?

Anger is real. Persistent, unresolved anger helps no one and can lead to depression and social problems. You must come to understand what you are angry about and then take steps to dissipate the anger. One way for believers to help resolve anger is through the power of Reinhold Niebuhr's serenity prayer:

> God, grant me serenity
> to accept the things I cannot change
> courage to change the things I can
> and the wisdom to know the difference

In addition, it will help if you learn to

- accept that many people do not understand what you need at this time and to appreciate it when their intentions are good
- sacrifice some comforts, opportunities, and hopes, at least for the time being, until your life is more settled (be willing to decline party invitations, job offers, or hobby-related outings that would overtax your emotional and physical reserves)
- share your anger in a safe place
- express your anger in writing, singing, drawing, music, or other medium
- accept yourself with your anger; accept yourself with any things you did in the past that may be making you angry; take responsibility for managing your anger

Unresolved anger does not help anyone and can lead to depression and social problems.

What If I Feel Sad?

Sadness is a feeling of unhappiness. Disappointment, grief, fatigue, and loneliness can all cause you to feel sad. Contrary to what people expect, you may experience your most intense sadness after treatment is completed.

Sadness may stem from disappointment in yourself or others at how things were handled during your treatment or how things are going now. One way many people get through the stresses and discomforts of cancer treatment is to focus on how good things will be when the treatment is over. If your life after cancer is a far cry from the inspirational, idealized images on which you focused during your treatments, you inadvertently set yourself up for disappointment once your treatment has ended.

Another critical reason for this posttreatment sadness is grief. After the intensity and routine of cancer treatments are over, you are left with all of your big and little losses to grieve. You may have lost

- your illusion of good health and safety
- a body part, such as a breast, a limb, or your voice
- a bodily function, such as mobility or fertility
- your normal energy
- time that you had planned to use doing something other than treat cancer
- the predictability of some relationships
- your appetite, your enjoyment of food
- your normal appearance
- insurance
- financial security
- expected opportunities at work, in school, or socially

What Is Grief?

The human reaction to loss is grief—a heavy feeling in the chest, mental distress, and a sense of emptiness and sadness. We all grieve our losses in order to process them and move forward in a healthy way. Denying your losses, or not allowing yourself to grieve adequately, deprives you of the comfort and relief that come from healthy grieving.

If I Am Experiencing Loss(es), How Should I Grieve?

First, figure out what it is you are grieving. Acknowledge the losses, and express your feelings about the losses. It is best to share your feelings of loss with someone who can understand you, validate your feelings, and comfort you.

People unfamiliar with issues of recovery may not be supportive. They are liable to say things like "Don't worry about your missing breast; at least you're alive" or "Don't worry about your girlfriend leaving you; if she left, she wasn't much of a girlfriend anyway." Your losses are real losses, and must be grieved. Lesser losses than death still need to be grieved. Having faced a life-threatening illness did not make you immune to the pain of losses.

Express your feeling of loss through art, music, or writing. If you feel like crying, cry. Find a safe place where you can cry freely.

There is no pill or magic that lets you bypass the grieving process. It takes time and expression.

Take comfort in the knowledge that experiencing the pain of your grieving will enable you to move forward and recapture joy and excitement.

What If I Feel Depressed?

Depression is a state of emotional dejection and withdrawal. It is marked by

- sadness
- loss of self-confidence
- change in appetite
- change in sleeping pattern
- fatigue
- loss of libido
- loss of interest
- loss of ability to concentrate
- somatic complaints such as a headache or stomachache

Depression after completion of cancer therapy can be due to or worsened by

- chronic pain
- chronic fatigue
- sleep deprivation
- medications
- hormonal imbalance
- chemical imbalance
- emotional stress

• feelings of helplessness
• resurfacing of old, unresolved problems
• loss of self-esteem
• unresolved grief or anger
• flare up of an underlying mood disorder

Depression is a symptom, like pain or nausea. Although a positive attitude and a solid faith can often help prevent or offset depression, they cannot always do so. Depression indicates that something is wrong, not necessarily that something is wrong with the way you are handling your situation.

Some women who have uneventful pregnancies and deliveries, and who are prepared and thrilled to receive this addition to their family, suffer from depression after they get home. This so-called postpartum depression is believed to be due to the effect on their brain of the drastic chemical and hormonal changes following delivery. Not all new mothers get depressed. Not all new mothers with depression are suffering from postpartum depression; some may have good reason to be depressed (the pregnancy was not wanted, the baby is not well, and so on). But it helps women who do suffer from genuine postpartum depression to learn that the depression is real, is due to chemical and hormonal changes beyond their control, is not due to their having a bad attitude or adjusting poorly, and is treatable.

Most cancer survivors have legitimate reasons to feel depressed (losses, strains, ongoing problems). However, depression can persist even after the survivor has grieved losses, accepted limitations, and resolved problems. Even if you have an ideal positive attitude and exceptional coping skills, the physical changes caused by chronic stress and/or the aftereffects of treatment may increase the risks of your becoming depressed. Thankfully, this depression usually responds well to treatment (medications and/or counseling). Understanding the physical nature of depression will spare you unnecessary suffering from this treatable aftereffect.

If you feel depressed, remember that you may be doing everything right to maximize your recovery from cancer treatment and yet have undergone physical changes that cause persistent depression. Similarly, someone with diabetes can take every measure to keep his blood sugar under control, can be very well adjusted to the changes and limitations required by his disease, and may nevertheless still need insulin, because his chemistry has been changed by the loss of insulin-producing cells.

Among the many different types of depression are manic-depressive disorder, major unipolar depression, and seasonal affective disorder (SAD). It is important that your doctor evaluate your depression because an accurate diagnosis increases the chance of revealing a reversible cause and beginning effective treatment.

What Should I Do If I Feel Depressed?

As stated above, depression is a symptom that signals that something is wrong and needs attention. First, find out why you are depressed, by discussing your feelings with your doctor. He or she needs to make sure that there is no medical reason for your depression. While evaluation is under way, your doctor may offer medication for short-term relief.

Second, be sure to get adequate rest and nutrition, even if it means temporarily taking some additional medication to improve appetite or sleep. Even when your depression is not due to sleep deprivation or malnutrition, good rest and nutrition will help you overcome the depression. In addition, appropriate exercise can help you feel proactive and in control, as well as cause physical changes that help lift your spirits.

Third, try to find positive things that have come out of your experiences with cancer, and focus on them.

Fourth, get some professional counseling to help you sort out the causes for your depression and find ways to work through the depression. Most people can get through periods of depression without professional counseling, but it usually shortens their duration, makes them less lonely and painful, and promotes emotional growth from which you benefit for the rest of your life.

If you have thoughts of harming yourself, or if you feel that everything would be easier if you just didn't wake up ever again, share this with your family, friends, or doctor. Destructive or suicidal thoughts are your mind's way of telling you that you need assistance to get back on the road to health. Getting help shows strength and gives added meaning to having survived your cancer.

What Good Can Come out of Having Cancer?

Although no reasonable person would desire to have cancer, many good things can come out of the cancer experience. After you have had a chance to absorb and process many of the changes, your having survived cancer can offer you

- a new, more balanced perspective on your life and your world. Insignificant problems will cause you less grief. Small pleasures will be savored with a new appreciation.
- an increased ability to feel empathy and compassion for others. This will enable you to better recognize and respond to their needs.
- a recognition of strong relationships that have stood the test of "for better or for worse." These relationships will be deeper and more precious for having grown through your cancer experience.
- the energizing and clarifying power of the sense of "a second chance."
- the opportunity for the deep expression and sharing of love and caring. Surviving cancer can break down barriers to meaningful communication.
- cherished, life-enhancing memories of people who provided support and help. A more optimistic view of our world is often a consequence of your life's having been touched by hospital staff and volunteers, support group participants, neighbors, and strangers who showed they cared.
- a deep, inner peace that is often seen in people who have gone through the stages of grief before dying. Having looked death in the eye and survived, you will have longer to appreciate this peace and to let it shape your life.
- a new meaning and direction to your life. Cancer often helps people find a new purpose in their life.

- a deeper respect for your emotional courage and spiritual strength. "If I could get through cancer, I can get through other challenges."
- a set of tools for living well that allows you to avoid or solve non-cancer-related problems.

What If I Feel Lonely?

Completing intensive therapy may feel like returning to earth from another planet. It is common to feel that most of the people around you do not really understand where you have been or where you are now. You may feel unsure of your responsibilities, your role, or even your identity. You are not your precancer self, you are no longer a full-time or part-time cancer patient, and you are not yet feeling normal. You are living in limbo.

You have left the security of organized, predictable, frequent medical attention. Even though you did not like being poked and prodded for all your evaluations and treatments, these inconveniences were accompanied by companionship and support. All that individual attention ended abruptly with your last treatment.

Your family, friends, co-workers, and acquaintances may feel awkward trying to relate to you now that your treatments are over. You step in the elevator and greet longtime acquaintances. They say hello and then look from their shoes to the elevator numbers to the walls and back to their shoes. Not wanting to say the wrong thing, and not knowing what to say, they say nothing. Simple interchange that you use to confirm your sense of belonging is strained, feeding your sense of loneliness.

After dealing with serious medical and emotional issues, you may feel uncomfortable or impatient with others' relatively mundane conversation. It is especially lonely when you feel that you no longer fit into your old world but that you do not yet have a new world to replace that of being a cancer patient. Take comfort in knowing that you will fit in again with time.

The bottom line is that you went through treatment and faced a life-threatening illness yourself. No matter how much love and support you feel, you are the one facing your illness, your fears, and your future.

One of the hardest aspects of completing treatment is that the average observer seems to expect you to feel only relief and joy. The average person does not recognize the stress of completing therapy. You may keep your fears and anxieties to yourself to avoid sounding ungrateful or pathologically depressed. Surviving your personal challenge of cancer can be very lonely.

What Can I Do If I Feel Lonely?

Surviving cancer is lonely only as long as you keep other people shut out of your world. Take the time and energy to explain to the people close to you how you feel and what you are thinking. The people who care about you are not mind readers. Dealing with your survival is new territory for them as well as for you, and they need your input to know how best to relate to you and how to help you. Be sure they understand that you are not necessarily sharing your problems and feelings in order for them to fix things. Just having an understanding, sympathetic ear is comforting and healing.

If you believe that there are absolutely no people out there who could possibly understand how you feel, then you have not connected yourself with cancer survivors farther along the road to recovery. Many survivors understand what you have been through and how you feel now. Many appreciate the chance to share and help. They can help you in a way that the most well-intentioned, loving, and thoughtful people who have not experienced cancer cannot. Now is a good time to find out about support groups, hotlines, and one-on-one matched support people such as the American Cancer Society's "CanSurmount" if you did not pursue this during your cancer therapy. Some cancer survivors wait years to try a support group, having lived with loneliness, fear, and anger for an unnecessarily long time.

If you feel lonely, reach out to others.

What If I Feel That I Have Little Control over My Life?

You lost your sense of control over your well-being when you were diagnosed with cancer. Throughout your treatment the only real control you had over your health was choosing to follow your treatment team's schedule and demands. Now that treatment is done, you are in the never-never land of "wait and see." Just as you could not protect yourself from your cancer when you were diagnosed, you cannot guarantee that you will be free of medical problems in the future.

Normal, everyday events that represent lack of control can be blown up out of proportion because of an underlying sensitivity to things you cannot control. Everyone deals with car breakdowns, leaky faucets, missed appointments, delayed flights, or sprained ankles. During recovery from cancer treatment, these ordinary setbacks can take on greater emotional meaning, because they tap into sensitivity about not having control. Your frustration at your lack of control over a delayed flight can unleash your frustration at your inability to have complete control over your cancer. In addition, you may have fewer reserves for dealing with problems and inconveniences. When you are well rested, you can clean up an overflowed sink and still have energy left over. When you are fatigued, the job may deplete your remaining energy.

When little setbacks occur because of treatment-related handicaps, your reaction may be exaggerated. Overflowing your bathtub or being late picking up your child from school is upsetting enough. You may feel worse when these things happen because you fell asleep from exhaustion.

If I Feel That Everything Is Out of Control, How Can I Regain a Sense of Control?

You have a certain need to control things in your life. Some people want and need the sense of a lot of control; others do not have as strong a need. You can regain a healthy sense of control by

- recognizing when you are associating lack of control over something minor with lack of control over your health
- limiting your commitments until you have the reserves to handle them all
- reminding yourself that minor problems are minor (you know what major problems are; draw attention to the insignificance of minor hassles)

The serenity prayer provides comfort and guidance when dealing with issues of control.

What Is "Checkup Anxiety"?

Checkup anxiety is the experiencing of anxiety, irritability, sleep disturbance, or increased somatic symptoms prior to a routine checkup. A man who was treated successfully for lung cancer gets chest pain a few weeks before every annual checkup. His pain gets worse as the checkup approaches and disappears after his test results document his continued remission. Another survivor, who is usually confident about his continuing good health, has a rough few days before every checkup. He has nightmares and daymares about getting bad news, and he is short-tempered and somewhat irrational.

There are many reasons for checkup anxiety. The obvious one is your fear that the checkup will reveal recurrent cancer. Other factors contribute to checkup anxiety:

- You have to reenter the realm of patient.
- Even the most well-suppressed memories of your cancer experience are rejuvenated somewhere between the fasting the night before, the waiting room filled with patients, the blood tests and X rays, and the interactions with uniformed doctors and nurses.
- You know that in the time it takes to relay your test results, your world can go from normality to chaos.
- Those around you may be anxious about your checkup, thus straining relationships and making you more anxious.

• You may have to juggle your checkup with other responsibilities, which just creates more stress.
• You feel out of control when you are being evaluated.

If I Am Experiencing Checkup Anxiety, What Can I Do to Minimize It?

The best cure for checkup anxiety is a series of normal checkups. Until that time, you can minimize checkup anxiety with some practiced attitudes and habits:

• Treat checkups as just one more necessary part of your life, like getting gas for your car or locking all the doors and windows before you leave your house.
• See checkups as an opportunity to confirm that you are doing well. You will feel great after you find out that your tests look good.
• Plan a special treat for yourself for soon after your checkup. Whenever you start to feel anxious, visualize yourself enjoying your special treat in the same way that you anticipate other planned, special happy events.
• After each checkup, fulfill the planned special treat. Reinforce the experience of good checkups. Make checkups something to look forward to, something associated with great memories.

One young mother who had intensive chemotherapy used to go to a department store after each treatment to buy something special. "Doesn't treatment mean you are meant (ment) for a treat?" she asks. She jokes with her friends that she is still paying off her medical *and* her department store bills from her treatments. She continues to do something special after each checkup and to joke about her department store bills. It can be an inexpensive treat, or just taking time to do or see something special. The key is a special reward to turn checkups into a celebration.

• See checkups as your opportunity to stay well. If you should develop a problem such as anemia, a recurrent cancer, a new

cancer, or a heart problem, regular checkups will maximize the
chance that your problem will be picked up early, when it is
most easily curable and has the least impact on your life.

• Remind yourself that if your checkup is going to reveal a problem, you want to know it. If you should develop a problem, you
will have it whether you go for your checkup or not. Avoiding
your checkups just delays when it is picked up and may
decrease your chance for some treatment options or even a cure.

You may play mind games while waiting for your checkup.
Should you hope that everything is perfect? Should you plan on
it? Are you confident that all is well, or do you have doubts?
Should you picture your doctor calling you to say that all of your
test results are great and not allow yourself to indulge in negative
fantasies? Or should you make plans for good news or bad news?

There is no one right way to play the waiting game. Some
approaches work well for some people and not for others. The
same approach may work well for you one time and not another.
In general, try to find the way that requires the least energy to
bring you the most comfort.

You may feel best assuming that everything will be perfect and
not letting yourself entertain for a minute any other possibility.
You may prefer planning for every contingency, going through all
possible outcomes in your mind and working through a plan of
action for each. You may find it easiest to prepare for bad news,
just like some smart people who go into every test saying, "I'm
going to fail," before they ace it. Or you may be able to put it out
of your mind entirely until you go.

**Checkups offer opportunities to confirm that you are doing
well, to stay well, and to celebrate your life.**

What If I Am Highly Emotional during the Holidays?

Holidays mark time and serve as the backdrop for important
memories. They also provide an opportunity to express feelings
that we are usually too busy or too self-conscious to share. There-

fore it is not surprising that holidays may precipitate strong emotions after completion of cancer treatment.

During the holidays you are bombarded by clichés and sayings found in greeting cards and in holiday songs. After your cancer experience sentiments like "Being with you is all that matters" or "I am happy to have today" trigger strong emotions, because they are meaningful and personal in a new way.

Thoughts about how the holiday might have been had your cancer not responded to treatment may be mixed with thoughts of how it might have been had you never gotten cancer in the first place. You may wonder how many holidays you have left to celebrate. You grieve for what you did lose, what you could have lost, and what you may still lose.

Although the treatment period may have been a blur, you can probably remember how your cancer affected this holiday during your treatment and thus be reminded of a time that you might prefer to forget.

Expect strong emotions on holidays. Let every holiday be a celebration of your life and what you do have.

What Is an "Anniversary Reaction"?

People often develop symptoms or emotions around the time of the anniversary of an event. Consciously and subconsciously, anniversary dates of births, deaths, weddings, divorces, accidents, and traumas such as theft or rape rekindle deep emotions.

After cancer you have new anniversaries, such as that of your diagnosis, that of completing treatment, and that of a bone marrow transplant that was a lifesaver. The anniversary reaction can consist of any combination of feelings of anxiety, overwhelming gratitude, weepiness, sense of dislocation, exultation, and depression.

Common symptoms that occur around anniversaries include generalized anxiety, melancholy, sleeplessness, and irritability. People can also develop specific symptoms that may or may not be related to the anniversary event. An irritative cough may develop around the anniversary of a lung cancer diagnosis. Fatigue may develop around the anniversary of a bone marrow transplant. Friction between you and your spouse may develop near the anniversary of your diagnosis.

What Can Be Done about the Anniversary Reaction?

Recognize it as a conscious and subconscious remembering of an important event. Marvel at the complexity and intricacy of human behavior. Try to make it a "good" anniversary by focusing on the good aspects of where you are. Accept yourself if this is a difficult time for you. Arrange your schedule to accommodate your reactions, or schedule activities to distract you from unpleasant feelings. One family that survived the devastation of hurricane Andrew in 1992 made plans to see a big baseball game on the anniversary date in order to distract themselves from the memory of that terrifying experience. If you recognize what is happening, it will be less unsettling and you can plan for it in whatever way works best for you.

If you catch yourself reliving in your mind the original event of an unpleasant anniversary, train yourself to stop this counterproductive rumination. Think of something else, something positive and life affirming. On the anniversary of your diagnosis, do not dwell on the details of being told. Do not relive the drama in your mind. Reliving bad experiences, even if only in memory, revives the associated feelings. It is best to reinforce positive, good feelings.

See anniversaries as opportunities to reinforce good feelings about your life.

What If I Can't Stop Thinking about My Cancer?

You may be wondering when you will go a week, a day, or even an hour without being reminded of your cancer experience. The more physical and/or social reminders you have of that experience, the harder it is to forget.

Physical pain and cancer treatment–related limitations are constant reminders until you reduce them to manageable levels and integrate them into your new life. Try to find some activities that capture your attention completely, no matter how briefly.

Cancer-related thoughts are triggered by insecurity about your renewed good health. You are ever vigilant for signs of a recurrence. It takes time to learn to trust your body again and enjoy your health.

You may have many unresolved feelings, such as anger, grief, disappointment, and depression, that are related to your cancer. Since these feelings will persist until the issues are resolved in one form or another, they remind you of your cancer. Attention to the feelings will liberate you from cancer-related thoughts.

A brush with mortality can make everything around you look and feel different. Since everything seems different, you are constantly reminded of why it seems so. Even when the changes and differences are good or pleasant, you are reminded of your cancer. With time you will get used to your new normal, and your surroundings will no longer remind you of your cancer.

It is fine to be reminded of your cancer if this elicits good feelings of gratitude and appreciation. If remembrance brings up unpleasant feelings such as anxiety, fear, and anger, you must work to resolve unsettled conflicts. You must also learn to look forward, not back.

It takes time to put a big event or experience out of your mind. Having some time and experiences unrelated to your cancer will help you stop thinking about your cancer.

Try to find good things that have come out of your cancer experience so that when you are reminded of your cancer, the feeling will not be all bad.

Is There Something Wrong with Me If I Don't Think about My Cancer?

As long as you are responsible about your posttreatment health care and follow-ups, it is great if you do not think about your cancer. If your cancer required relatively brief, easily tolerated therapy, if your prognosis is good, and if your cancer experience did not change your outlook on life, then it would be expected and healthy for you to forget about your cancer most of the time.

If you do not think about your cancer, because when you do you experience uncomfortable, even intolerable feelings, then you are repressing, not forgetting, memories of your cancer experience. It is best if your cancer history and cancer experience become integrated parts of your past.

What If I Miss Going for Treatment?

Inconvenient and uncomfortable as treatment may have been, it had its good sides:

- You had the comfort of knowing that you were doing something active to treat your cancer.
- You were the recipient of undivided attention.
- People were gentle and sympathetic toward you.
- You felt like everyone else at the doctor's office; outside the medical setting you may feel like the only cancer patient.

What Can I Do If I Miss Being a Patient?

Recognize the sources of your anxiety and allay it through knowledge, hope, and action. Savor the current success of your treatment, no matter how uncertain the future. Relish your liberation from treatments, visits, and tests.

You can replace the missing interactions by making efforts to get together with new people who understand your situation, needs, and emotions. Support groups and professional counseling can fill in some of the gaps during this transition to a new normal life.

If you find yourself wishing you were still a patient and reluctant to resume the interactions and responsibilities of healthy people, it may be helpful to reexamine the life you are reentering. Your illness may have functioned as a shield against unpleasant aspects of your everyday existence as a healthy person. Take stock of your values, priorities, and goals. Think about how your personal and professional pursuits do and do not satisfy you.

It is normal to miss some aspects of being a patient. However, if you wish you were still a patient, that is a signal to make changes in your circumstances or your relationships. This may be the time for you to confront issues that you avoided prior to your illness. Professional help is available if you need support and guidance during this period of readjustment.

What If I Feel Less Familiar with or Less Sure about My Body?

As you grow up, you learn the strengths and weaknesses of your body. By the time you are an adult, you know whether you are double-jointed or inflexible, a sprinter or a long-distance runner, resistant or susceptible to infections, mellow or hyperexcitable, a heavy or a light sleeper, a pessimist or an optimist "by nature," sensitive to foods or able to eat anything that doesn't walk, and so on.

Cancer and cancer therapy can upset patterns that have been set for a long time and have come to feel comfortable in identifying "you." Being different in a few or many ways is unsettling, especially if unexpected and undesired. You do not know what to expect of your body or emotions, so you do not know what the rules are any more. You have become unfamiliar with the body and emotions you always knew best—your own.

If before your episode with cancer all sore throats, coughs, headaches, stomachaches, or backaches cleared up by themselves if left alone, you learned that these things did not need medical attention or intervention. Now that you have had cancer and cancer therapy, some of these symptoms may signal a problem for you that needs early intervention to prevent a more serious illness. The same symptoms that you had before your cancer now have different implications. Depending on your type of cancer, your type of treatment, your medical condition before cancer, and your style of dealing with symptoms, you may need to become reacquainted with your body and learn a new style for dealing with its signals.

Bodily changes happen to all people as they get older, but they happen over decades. Gradual changes allow gradual acceptance and adaptation. Cancer and its treatment cause enormous changes practically overnight. Unfortunately, the acceptance and adaptation still take a long time. There is a disparity between how quickly the changes occurred and affected your life and how quickly you can absorb the changes and adjust. This disparity causes a sense of unfamiliarity and stress.

Is It Okay to Go to the Doctor for Every Little Lump or Cough?

If you develop a cough or a lump that concerns you, make an appointment to go to your doctor as soon as possible and have it evaluated. If you are not sure whether it needs evaluation, call your doctor's office for advice. You deserve to find out whether the problem needs attention or not. You deserve a speedy evaluation if the problem does warrant medical attention. Having a plan of action for problems will relieve everyone's anxiety before and when problems arise. The earlier you go for evaluation,

- the less time, energy, and emotion you will waste worrying about whether or not you should have it evaluated
- the less time you will have for your imagination to work on all the possible outcomes
- the less time a real problem will have to get serious

What If I Feel like a Hypochondriac?

A hypochondriac is someone who suffers from imaginary illnesses or problems. We use the term loosely to apply to anyone who seems overly concerned about his or her health.

After cancer, just as after a heart attack or after being treated for asthma, you are entitled to be a bit of a hypochondriac, especially in the first few months after therapy. It is adaptive and beneficial to you to be tuned in to your body's signals, especially when you are still adjusting to its changes.

Be safe, not sorry. It is better for you to call or see your doctors about a small problem and have them reassure you that it is nothing significant than to wait with a problem in order to avoid being considered a hypochondriac and end up with a more difficult problem to treat.

One survivor did not hesitate to put her family through the stress and expense of having her mild back pain evaluated. Another survivor tried to avoid the appearance of a hypochondriac, and to minimize her family's stress, by enduring a similar pain. The first survivor found out she had a pulled muscle and had it treated before there was any significant impact on her health or the family. The second woman got progressively worse. Her pulled muscle went into spasm, causing her to favor it and strain other muscles. The stress of worry caused her to develop an ulcer and her family relationships to become tense.

Doctors expect patients who have had cancer to be tuned in to their bodies and to be more concerned about common symptoms than a person who has never had cancer. Do not worry about being a hypochondriac. Do the right thing: listen to your body, and get yourself checked.

What If I Feel That My Body Has Failed Me?

In your mind, your body has failed you by allowing you to get cancer. Most of your friends did not get cancer. No matter how many wonderful skills your body demonstrated before, during, or after your cancer, pride in your body can be lost in the reality that your body got cancer.

Has My Body Really Failed Me?

Failure is a subjective conclusion. If you believe that nobody should get cancer, you will probably feel that your body failed you. However, if you realize that cancer has been threatening human life for millennia, you will see cancer as one of the potential threats for all people, along with infections and accidents.

Rather than failing you, your body sustained you despite the threat of cancer and the risks of cancer therapy. Your body overcame a challenge it did not want and for which it did not prepare.

You are surviving. Instead of blaming your body for getting cancer, congratulate it for surviving cancer and its treatment.

Is It Common to Feel like Damaged Goods?

Many cancer survivors feel that they are damaged goods. The so-called damage may be painfully obvious, such as loss of voice, fertility, limb, speech, breast, continence, or sexual function. In other cases the losses are subtle or invisible to the outside observer, such as lost stamina, spontaneity, self-esteem, or confidence in the future.

You may look and feel perfectly normal and yet still see yourself as damaged goods. After all, you have had cancer and could develop it again. The knowledge that some cancer patients have a genetic predisposition to their and other cancers may just reinforce your self-perception of being damaged goods.

Future health risks are not unique to cancer survivors. All people have their risk factors, be it their risk for stroke, heart attack, emphysema, rheumatoid arthritis, kidney disease, or manic-depressive disorder. Cancer survivors can learn to see cancer as just one of the risk factors they need to consider in their health maintenance and preventive medicine measures.

Loss and change, too, are not unique to cancer survivors. Many diseases are accompanied by loss and change. You are no more damaged than someone with a history of heart disease or lupus. Quite often the quality of life and prognosis for someone with heart disease or lupus is worse than for someone with many types of cancer. In our society, still, the word "cancer" carries stronger connotations of suffering and death than the words "heart disease" or "lupus."

Nobody is perfect. To be normal is to be flawed.

If I Feel Like Damaged Goods, How Can I Feel "Whole" Again?

Feeling whole is a state of mind. If you see yourself as whole, you are whole. An important means to this end is to recognize what makes you "you." Your essence goes far beyond job, clothes size, and talents. Self-reflection, discussion with family, friends, support people and groups, and professional counseling can help you discover or rediscover who you are.

If you have suffered a loss that strips you of your livelihood, hobbies, or usual means of communication or mobilization, you may have to change your definition of yourself. Your losses may allow you to see and develop strengths and abilities you never appreciated or knew you had.

If you have sustained a physical loss, there are healthy ways to adjust and compensate:

- Gather facts. Find out as much as you can about treatment options for your problem.
- Find out whether surgery or mechanical devices are available to repair or compensate for the lost part or function.
- If the loss is permanent, learn as much as you can about how to cope with it. Find support groups specific to your needs. No matter how devastating your physical losses, other people have experienced the same losses and have learned ways to integrate the losses and get on with their lives. Seek out these people for practical advice and sympathetic support.
- Expect to grieve your losses for some period of time before you learn to accept and adapt to them. It often takes time and hard work.

It takes more energy to find a way to be happy and fulfilled despite your circumstances than to be unhappy. The rewards are invaluable for you and your family.

Emphasize all the new insights and strengths you have gained from your cancer experience. Your priorities and sensitivities have been shaped by powerful forces. As Nietzsche said, "What does not kill you makes you strong."

You cannot choose the changes and losses that accompanied your cancer. You can choose how these changes and losses shape your life.

Is It Common to Feel Old Suddenly?

Many of the physical symptoms experienced soon after cancer treatment are similar to those, rightly or wrongly, associated with old age, such as fatigue, decreased mental clarity, increased sleep requirements, and decreased appetite. Many of the insights you have acquired through your experiences may also make you feel older and wiser.

How Can I Transcend My Cancer Experience If I Have So Many Physical Reminders?

If you cannot change the physical scars of your experience with cancer, you need to redefine them in such a way that they represent something positive in your life. Cancer survivors can learn to see their physical and emotional scars as badges of courage and accomplishment.

How you feel about your cancer and yourself depends on your state of mind, not body.

What If I Am Anxious about the Health of Myself and My Family?

You have been burned once. You no longer feel safe. You underwent a crisis. You feel that it can happen to someone you love. It is very common to be anxious about your health and that of your family for a while after completing treatment. When you feel well again and have gained some distance from the treatment experience, this anxiety will fade. For some people the anxiety resolves completely. For others it almost resolves but resurfaces easily in the face of any symptom, change, or threat. If this anxiety persists unabated, it must be addressed.

Instead of worrying about how anxious you are, do something about it. Find out quickly whether something is worth worrying about, by getting it checked out. Do not waste your energy trying not to be anxious or worrying that you are being overanxious. You deserve not to have to worry so much. The doctor bills for a problem that turns out to need no treatment may have been avoidable from a medical point of view, but it is worth it for you to be saved some anxiety. If your doctor reassures you that there is no significant problem, be grateful. You cannot know ahead of time which things are going to turn out okay and which are real problems. Remind yourself that you deserve to not worry.

What Can I Do to Be Less Anxious about My Health?

You can take a number of steps to diminish your anxiety about your health:

- Be informed about your follow-ups.
- Know the signs and symptoms for which you should see your doctor.
- Learn about all proven ways to maximize your health and minimize your chance of recurrence.
- Be in tune with your body, recognizing when something is a signal to you that medical attention is needed.
- Be willing to call your doctor when you suspect that something is wrong.
- Recognize and accept that you cannot control everything. You cannot control every exposure to food, radiation, additives, pollution, or emotional stress.

What If I Feel Like a Young Child Sometimes?

After completion of cancer treatment you are physically and emotionally vulnerable. Your physical and emotional needs are greater than they were before your cancer. Under the best of circumstances, you still need help, attention, support, and comfort.

You may experience this vulnerability and neediness as something embarrassing to yourself and to others. Neediness may be confused with immaturity or weakness. Your vulnerability is an expected consequence of the treatment. Your neediness is the normal, healthy consequence of recognized vulnerability.

Just as thirst protects you from dehydration, neediness protects you from isolation that would be detrimental to your physical and emotional well-being. Respect your neediness as your well-balanced self attending to itself. You feel needy because after cancer treatment you have legitimate needs. Satisfying these needs will encourage uneventful healing, physically and emotionally.

What If I Find Myself Reacting like a Child to Stresses?

Children are expected to have little tolerance for stress. When a two-year-old licks the scoop of ice cream off the cone and onto the floor, the expected, normal response is to cry. The two-year-old child cries from disappointment, frustration, and a sense of powerlessness.

Losing a scoop of ice cream will elicit some emotions at any age, but will be less and less likely to cause you to cry as you get older. As an adult, you have acquired a repertoire of feelings, thoughts, and actions that allows you to absorb and respond to stresses in a socially acceptable way. You developed these tools as you matured and practiced them until they became your normal way of responding. Mature responses give you identity and self-respect.

During recovery from cancer treatment you may find yourself literally crying after little stresses like that of losing your ice cream. When you are under great stress, especially chronically, you may temporarily lose access to some of your acquired mature responses. This state is called regression, where you feel and act like a child in stressful situations that, under more normal circumstances, you would handle in a mature way.

Cancer survivors can experience regression during recovery because of

- fatigue
- anxiety
- sleep deprivation
- pain
- frustration
- medications
- effect of the cancer or cancer treatment on the brain

Extra emphasis needs to be given to the effect of sleep deprivation and fatigue. These two factors have a major impact on how we see and react to the world around us, and they are the easiest two to control.

Regression is a normal response to chronic physical and emotional stress. Although you may find it embarrassing or frustrating, regression is a mechanism of self-protection that helps you attend to your needs and conserve your energy.

What Can I Do about My Responding like a Child?

When you feel and see yourself responding like a child, it will help to

- accept this as a common, normal, temporary part of recovery
- accept yourself with your human needs
- get extra rest
- avoid unnecessary stresses
- let your support people know what things are difficult for you and what things help

Understandably, serious illness can cause you to become preoccupied with yourself, another characteristic often associated with children. A degree of self-centeredness after cancer treatment is necessary for healing, because it allows you to recognize your physical and emotional needs and conserve your energy for recuperation.

What If News of Someone Else's Death from Cancer Makes Me Highly Emotional?

Hearing of someone else's death from cancer forces you to remember that cancer, including your cancer, can be a life-threatening disease. It is difficult to function, let alone enjoy life, if you are constantly thinking about your mortality. During treatment one of the ways you control your thoughts about mortality is to focus on your treatments. After treatment, as you begin to feel safe again, you may calm your anxiety by rethinking your recent past: "I wasn't in real danger when I was sick. It was scary, but I was going to do okay, and I would do okay if I developed cancer again." You tame thoughts about the life-threatening nature of cancer by seeing your disease as a chronic illness that requires treatments. It is adaptive and healthy to see yourself as having a disease with which you can live.

Whenever you learn about another's death, whether you have had cancer or not, it disturbs your sense of being safe from death. This uneasiness is greater if the person was of similar age or social circumstance. It is extreme when the possibility of your own death is more real for your having faced it. Past and present fears that you successfully suppressed during and after your cancer treatment come to the surface, making you anxious or afraid.

To deal with the emotions, remember that another person's death has no affect on whether or when you will die. You may be worried, consciously or subconsciously, that if someone else succumbed from cancer, then you will. Many factors determine what happens with your cancer. Someone else's course and outcome tell you nothing about your future course and outcome. Even if you hear of a series of people who die from the same type of cancer that you had, remember that they were all different people in different circumstances.

You may worry that someone's death affects the statistics about your prognosis. It does not. Consider an analogy: If you flip a coin, you have a fifty-fifty chance of landing it on heads. If you do it four times, and each time you get heads, then the fifth time you still have a fifty-fifty chance (assuming, of course, that it is not a trick coin).

For each coin flip the prognosis of getting heads is fifty-fifty, no matter what the results of the other flips. Similarly, your prognosis is independent of everyone else's. If statistics say that 80 percent of all people with your cancer survive five years, someone else's death does *not* increase or decrease your chance of surviving. It is not as if, by someone else's being one of the 20 percent who succumb, you have more of a chance of being in the 80 percent surviving.

On the other hand, your being in the 80 percent of the people who are surviving did not hurt the other person's chance of surviving. You could affect someone else's prognosis only if there was just enough treatment for one of you, and you got it.

You may feel guilty that you survived, especially when the other person was younger than you, fought his or her cancer at the same time that you fought yours, or appeared to deal with the disease better. This is called survivor's guilt, and it is seen in survivors of disasters. The thought "Why did I survive when she didn't?" taps into emotional issues like the meaning of your life. You may feel a rush of gratitude that you are alive, and then feel guilty that you were happy for yourself when someone else died. Being relieved that it was not you does not hurt anyone and in no way means you are glad someone else died.

Another reason that news of someone's else death from cancer can touch you deeply is that you have a better sense of what that person went through before he or she died.

If you knew the person fairly well, you may remember hearing the words "I know I can beat this." We all want to believe that we can use will power to make things turn out a certain way. Whenever you hear someone sound confident about surviving, you want to believe it, for that person as well as for yourself.

It is unsettling when someone with a positive attitude dies, especially if you think that death signifies the failure of a positive attitude. The benefit of a positive attitude is to be judged not only in terms of survival but also in terms of the quality and, possibly, the length of life. If someone with a positive attitude dies, you can be assured that his or her quality of life was better during life than it would have been without that attitude. And maybe he or she lived longer too. A positive attitude is a major asset no matter what the ultimate outcome.

How Can I Deal with Other People's Cancer Death?

To grieve when you have to deal with another's death is normal. This has not changed just because you, too, had cancer. Preparing for someone's death or understanding the source of your feelings will not keep you from having feelings when the person dies. You must allow yourself to go through the grieving process, even if it means touching on some feelings that are discomfitting. Unthinking, unfeeling people are protected from the pain of grief. Accept your feelings as a sign of your personal depth and your connection with the world.

Talk about the person and your feelings. Allow yourself to cry, feel mellow, or be distracted and inefficient for a while. Remember that some of your emotions may seem a little bit out of proportion, because the news may have stirred up emotions about issues that are closer to you. The loss of a casual friend from cancer can awaken major grief over other losses, as well as your own fears.

Remind yourself that death is not defeat. Death is a normal, natural, unavoidable, expected part of life. Living the life you have is a victory. Someone can die with chemotherapy dripping, fighting cancer to the last breath, while someone else dies peacefully at home after accepting that the time to die has come. The act of choosing how to live your life is a triumph, no matter what the outcome.

What If I Feel Differently about Reading the Obituaries?

If you read the obituaries before your cancer diagnosis, reading them now is just the continuation of an old habit that satisfies certain needs for you. You may find the stories in the obituaries interesting. If you tend to check the age and cause of death, you are satisfying a somewhat morbid curiosity common to many people. It helps some to keep the perspective that life is short and not to be wasted.

If you never read the obituaries before your cancer diagnosis and now catch yourself reading them, it can be an uncomfortable, anxiety-provoking, and embarrassing self-revelation. Reading obituaries is a common behavior after cancer treatment, with many possible roots. Part of you wants to deny your recent brush with a life-threatening disease. To balance your denial and reach a realistic yet comfortable balance, you read the obituaries. This allows the other side of you to reassert that you are mortal and that many people do die of cancer. This process takes place on a subconscious level.

Seeing reports of others' demise perhaps bolsters your sense of accomplishment when you are feeling low in other areas. "I survived. That is the important thing." Or perhaps you still find it so hard to grasp the enormity of your cancer experience that you look to the obituaries for some sense of reality. This is similar to looking at the wreckage of a car after an accident, as if by looking at the crumpled metal you could understand the event.

Should I Avoid Reading the Obituaries?

Do not worry about it. Do not give yourself more anxiety by worrying about your behavior. You do not have to control everything. If you feel like reading obituaries, read them. If it bothers you to read them, turn the page. If you dwell on the obituaries and cannot stop thinking about death, get some professional help to sort out your fears and feelings.

What If Old Emotionally Charged Problems Unrelated to My Cancer Have Resurfaced?

Completion of cancer therapy is an emotional time, with anxiety, sadness, anger, and other emotions all stirred up. This setting of high emotions often triggers recall of past events or problems that elicited similar emotions that were never well resolved.

You may not have adequately grieved the premature loss of a parent or sibling. After completion of your cancer therapy, as you deal with grief over loss of a body part or loss of a job, you may reexperience a deep sense of loss of your parent or sibling.

Many problems and issues that were important before your diagnosis became dwarfed by the immediacy of your cancer and its treatment. Since the problems were not resolved, but rather forced into the background, they can reappear after treatment. These problems can be even more complicated and pressing after cancer because of the changes in your life. If before you had cancer you and your spouse argued about the amount of time and money you spent on leisure activities, or about the division of labor at home, these arguments can resurface with an added edge of urgency.

Problems pop up periodically for everyone, even in families that are not dealing with cancer or other crisis. Resist the temptation to blame every bad and unpleasant thing, every change and adjustment, on your cancer. Instead of using your cancer as a focus of blame, you should use it as a reminder that you can get through hard times.

Your cancer experience is not responsible for everything difficult or unpleasant that arises after cancer. Normal life involves good and bad times, easy and hard times, tense and relaxed times, happy and sad times.

What Can I Do If Emotions Are Surfacing in Regard to Past Issues?

See your unwanted cancer experience as an opportunity to put closure on lingering or reappearing unresolved issues. Your survival of cancer can show you that, with proper help and guidance, you now have the tools and strength to deal with these old issues.

Emotions do not go away by themselves. They go away when the problems that precipitated them are resolved or coped with in a healthy way. If you try to ignore or deny your emotions or the causative issues, they will continue to affect you in negative ways. In the long run it takes less physical and emotional energy to resolve than to deny problem emotions and issues.

One couple was very stressed by the wife's loss of employment. The husband felt that she could be doing more to find an acceptable job. The two were reaching a point of confrontation when she developed cancer. The job issue became a nonissue. After completion of treatments the job issue resurfaced with a vengeance. The money concerns were obvious. The husband genuinely wanted to do what was right for his wife's recovery, but did not want to allow her to use her recent illness as an excuse for continuing the posture she had assumed before. A difficult issue became complicated by the overlay of the illness.

This couple's problem predated the cancer. With guidance the cancer history will not prevent the couple from dealing with this fundamental problem. Their approach to the problem and the possible solutions will be affected by the cancer experience. You can offset added difficulties by the insights and strengths you have acquired through surviving.

Strong emotions can signal unresolved problems or issues.

Do I Have to Deal with These Old Issues Now?

You do not have to deal with every problem at once, whether you have had cancer or not. You have to use judgment about which problems you can afford to postpone and which you can solve more easily with a little bit of distance. If your tax papers are out of order and you do not want to deal with them, but you will pay a heavy fine if you miss a filing date, the chore is probably worth getting done. If you have had strained relations with a relative who is moving far away or is terminally ill, and you think that you would like to mend things, now is the time. If you cannot decide what you want to major in at college, or you are thinking of changing careers, you can decide not to decide for a while.

The longer you delay dealing with a problem,

- the longer you will feel the negative effects
- the more energy you will be using to deal with the emotions and avoid dealing with the precipitating issue
- the greater the chance these old issues will have for creating new problems

Sometimes the intensity of your emotions in response to cancer-related issues is heightened by emotions about old issues that are being attributed to the cancer. Recognizing this will help you deal with the real issues and will make the cancer-related emotions much more manageable.

What If I Am Faced with Many Big Decisions in My Life Now That My Treatments Are Over?

Recovery from cancer treatment often brings opportunities for making big changes. Your work situation may have changed while you were being treated. Your changed perspective may lead you to feel that you want to make a career change. Plans to move may have been postponed, and now you feel differently about the move. An unhappy marriage that was tolerated for many years may now seem intolerable.

This is a wonderful time to think about making changes that will move you toward a more satisfying life at home and at work. You do not have to change or fix everything right away. Your top priority is getting well. On the other hand, you want to take advantage of windows of opportunity. You want to hold on to your changed perspective and priorities to create a better life.

You may be swept up in the emotional intensity of recovery, tempted to make major decisions that seem absolutely right at the time but that can hurt you in the long run. A woman built a successful accounting firm prior to her cancer diagnosis. After surviving eighteen months of rigorous treatments, she felt that she wanted to do something more meaningful with her life. She was ready to close her office, sell the equipment, and look for part-time work as a consultant for cancer-related causes. The glamour of her plan wore off, as she realized how profoundly her decision would affect her family's lifestyle and comfort and how she would lose the self-actualization that came from her flourishing accounting business. With time, she came to see her work as more meaningful. She provided an important service for others, and the contribution to the family income provided stability. Instead of abandoning her work, she made substantial changes in how she did it. Ultimately, she worked fewer hours per week, leaving more time for her children and volunteer work. Cancer encouraged her to look at what she was doing and make some positive changes in her life.

If you are going to undertake big changes or decisions, work with a close friend, family member, or professional counselor to arrive at wise, life-enhancing decisions. When possible, let some time pass before you make a final decision. Taking your time will help prevent rash decisions fueled by fear, anxiety, euphoria, fatigue, or stress. You want to look at alternatives in such a way that you do not hurt yourself professionally or financially. You must consider how any proposed changes will affect your family, insurance, health, and future job options.

How Do I Know Whether I Need Counseling?

Counseling is one way to help you deal with any stress or challenge. Through therapeutic listening and professional guidance, counseling provides support, understanding, and tools for making decisions about living your new life. Pursue counseling sooner rather than later if

- you are unable to communicate with your family and friends
- you are having trouble fulfilling your responsibilities
- you cannot sleep or eat
- you are unable to concentrate
- you feel overwhelmed
- you want professional guidance to maximize the benefits that can come from your cancer experience
- you feel that unresolved issues have resurfaced and need attention

Other signs that counseling might be beneficial include

- persistent anxiety
- depression
- persistent anger
- confusion

The surviving of cancer is hard work in uncharted territory. Getting help demonstrates strong survival instincts.

FEAR

What If I Feel Afraid?

On some level, you knew from the beginning of your treatment that if your cancer was not sensitive to the therapy, you could die from the cancer. You may even have joked about the harshness of your cancer treatments or your losses by saying, "The alternative is worse."

During treatment you focused on getting through the treatments and dealing with all the short-term practical issues. Now that the immediate risk of death by cancer is past, you may experience your underlying great fears. In an analogous situation a person is involved in a near-fatal car accident, survives because of level-headed defensive driving, and then walks away only to faint from fright after the danger is past. Or someone resuscitates a near-drowned child with calm and expertise and then falls to pieces as the now safe child is taken away.

You did what you had to do during your crisis of cancer. Now that your crisis is over, you acknowledge and experience the fear of your brush with death.

Fear of the unknown is common. Your future is a big unknown. The inability to know your future can cause fear, especially since you glimpsed potential futures when you learned about your cancer and saw other cancer survivors who were not doing well.

Fear can be a recurring emotion after you have been treated for cancer. It can take many forms—fear of recurrence, fear of death, fear of bodily injury or loss, fear of doctors, fear of financial hardship or ruin, and fear of embarrassment. Fear is paralyzing and painful. You must learn to recognize your fear, understand it, and tame it so that your cancer history does not define or control you.

How Do I Tame My Fears?

First, figure out what you are afraid of. Is it death, recurrence, future medical problems, rejection or abandonment by family (or friends, or co-workers, or health care workers), or financial problems? Second, share your fears with your family, friends, other cancer survivors, clergy, counselors, or support group.

Get information about the things you fear. Knowledge may

- eliminate fears that were based on misinformation
- allow you to maximize control over things you fear
- teach you a way to live with your fears

What If Many Questions, Fears, and Worries about My Cancer Have Resurfaced?

At the time you were first diagnosed, there were many questions, fears, and worries. Once the decisions about therapy were made and you began your treatment, you could put aside questions and concerns about the medium- and long-range future to some degree. After treatment you are again faced with many small and big decisions and uncertainties. You have to confront the reality of the changes that happened during treatment but that did not affect your life during treatment.

During treatment you may have had physical pain, but you focused on getting through your treatments. Having survived, you now fear ongoing or worsening pain.

If you are single and your treatment rendered you sterile, you may have been too ill during therapy to desire to socialize or worry about infertility. Now that you are getting well again, you may experience concern about the effect of your infertility on your social relationships. You may experience grief over your lost fertility now or later, even though the actual loss occurred during treatment.

Another source of renewed questions, fears, and worries is an insecurity that the posttreatment tests missed something. You may want reassurance that the treatments did indeed work and that they are all the treatments you will ever need. Even if everything goes perfectly and all your tests look good, the best you can be told is that you are fine right now. After treatment you reenter the world of judgment calls, multiple right choices, and great uncertainty.

How Can I Lessen These Worries?

The key to managing fears and worries is becoming informed and acting on your knowledge. Find out as much as you can about your situation, weigh all of your options, and then follow what feels right for you. After the decision has been made that no further therapy is needed, put all of your energy into getting and staying well.

There comes a time when you must trust the test results, trust your doctors, trust your decisions about therapy, and decide to put the issue behind you.

If you do not trust the test results or your decision that your therapy is complete, you need to find out why. Then pursue a route that will provide information and decisions that you can trust. If you feel that you will never trust any test results or any doctor's advice, it is time to speak with a counselor skilled in the issues of the cancer survivor.

In order to be emotionally healthy, you must be able to trust.

Is It Common to Have a Fear of Recurrence?

Almost all cancer survivors have some fear of recurrence. If you rarely think about your cancer or the possibility of recurrence, you are very lucky, as long as you are diligent with the advised follow-up for your cancer. If you are so confident of your continued cancer-free state that you skip advised checkups and tests, you are probably more afraid than confident. Delayed or missed checkups are missed opportunities to stay well.

Most cancer survivors harbor a certain fear of recurrence. For some it is a daily, debilitating fear. For most it is a repressed fear that surfaces only in the face of unavoidable reminders of vulnerability, such as checkups, anniversaries, a new pain, a cough, or a bump.

Fear of recurrence is a fear that can be managed.

Why Is the Fear of Recurrence So Intense?

The intensity of your fear reflects not how much you believe you could have a recurrence but what it is you fear. The fear of recurrence is very intense because of the impact of the meaning of recurrence, not necessarily because of how strongly you believe you will experience recurrence. People who are usually confident that they will stay well can experience intense fear under threatening circumstances, because the tiny shred of doubt touches on a deep and powerful fear.

Fear of recurrence can be more intense than fear of a first cancer. Most people who have not had cancer feel, on some level, that it could not happen to them. Even acknowledging that they know and believe that it could strike them tomorrow, a part of them feels safe. They have the adaptive, normal, healthy emotional protection of a sense of immunity.

Having had cancer, you know, intellectually and emotionally, that you really could develop cancer again. Cancer is no longer something that happens only to other people. It is easier to believe that you will never get cancer than to believe that you will never have a recurrence.

Fear of recurrence is powerful because you know what it is like to have cancer, to be a patient, to decide on treatment, and then to undergo treatment. You know too well that a cancer diagnosis involves job stress, family stress, financial stress, and inconvenience, at best, or great debility or death, at worst. You fear not just cancer but all the pain and losses that accompany it.

How Can I Manage My Fear of Recurrence?

Taming fear is one of the most important tasks you can tackle to help yourself and those around you after completion of cancer therapy. There are many ways to help tame your fear of recurrence. Some will help you more than others. Different things will help at different times. Find out which ways help you tame your fear. Some things that help include

- obtaining knowledge about your situation so that you do not worry about things that are not likely to happen
- obtaining information about how to minimize your chance of recurrence by modifying your diet, exercise, medications, and whatever else applies to your situation
- obtaining knowledge of how to participate in the surveillance of your condition (what things to look for that could indicate a problem)
- being willing to have potential problems evaluated
- distracting yourself from the fear by focusing on today and on things you enjoy
- accepting the reality that fearful thoughts will occur
- training yourself to shut off the fearful thoughts ("If I have a recurrence, I will deal with the circumstances at that time") or to distract yourself from fearful thoughts by thinking about something pleasant or neutral
- reminding yourself that recurrence is not a death sentence; that you were treated successfully before and can be treated successfully again; that although the idea of repeat cancer treatment may be overwhelming right now, you could handle it again if faced with recurrence; and that advances make cancer treatment more effective and tolerable every year
- ventilating your fears to appropriate others, such as cancer survivors, loved ones, clergy, or professional counselors

Fear will not help you today or tomorrow. Untamed fear ruins good times. The taming of fear frees you to live a better life.

What Can I Do to Decrease Any Fear That My Environment Is Putting Me at Risk for Recurrence?

Get knowledge about the real risk to you from your diet, work exposures, and home environment. Then take any steps you can to reduce your risk. Our current level of knowledge holds more questions than answers about the risk of diet and environmental exposures. Yesterday's advice is contradicted today, and today's advice is contradicted tomorrow. Advice that may help your cancer risk may increase risks of other medical problems. At this time a practical approach is to

- follow advice that has been well substantiated and has withstood the test of time
- make changes that do not involve too many adverse effects (do not allow yourself to get malnourished by dietary changes that are too restrictive)
- make changes that bring you reassurance and comfort, not anxiety and strain

What Can I Do to Decrease My Fear of Recurrence If It Is Based on the Statistics about My Type of Cancer?

Statistics can cause you to feel increased fear of recurrence, even if they are favorable. That is because statistics present you with a specific time frame and a scientific-sounding percentage, such as 85 percent survival in five years.

Learn to interpret information to your advantage. If the statistics and your doctors indicate that your risk of recurrence is small, believe them and assume that you will do as well as expected. Remind yourself repeatedly that you can expect to do well and that recurrence is not likely. If your risk of recurrence is great, remind yourself repeatedly that statistics do not say anything about how you in particular will do. Find something special about you or your cancer situation that sets you apart from the statistical mass. Remind yourself repeatedly that you can be the one who does well.

If this sounds contradictory and calculating, it is because healthy survivorship is a frame of mind. Being a healthy survivor means learning to process the information around you in a way that is adaptive for your unique situation. What is reassuring and strengthening for one survivor, such as survival statistics, can be detrimental to another. Use what works for you.

Just as facts should lead to action that diminishes fear, use them to create an attitude that diminishes your fear. Train yourself to reassure yourself in a genuine way. If you have ready responses for your fears, you will gain more and more control over your fears. Reminding yourself that you know what to do (second opinions, researching options, mobilizing support) if you should develop a recurrence will eliminate the component of fear that is due to the sense of being totally overwhelmed and out of control. Remind yourself of individuals who flourished after being treated for recurrent cancer or a type of cancer with a poor prognosis.

You cannot change the statistics regarding your cancer, but you can change how you interpret them and their impact on your life. Use statistics to help you.

Is There Any Way to Eliminate the Fear of Recurrence?

Most people can never completely eliminate the fear of recurrence. However, you can diminish your fear and make it very manageable. You can tame your fear in such a way that it has very little impact on your day-to-day life. Accepting that there will be times of fear and anxiety, and that these times will pass, helps disempower the fear and minimize its impact.

Recognize your fear for what it is—fear. Reassure yourself that it is natural and acceptable to have fear, and then reassure yourself that you can do things to lessen and control it.

What about Recurrence Scares?

Invariably, all cancer survivors suffer recurrence scares. A lump, a swollen arm, a backache, or a headache can trigger a cascade of thoughts that culminates in the fear of recurrence. This is a normal part of survivorship. You need to have a practiced plan of action of what to do and think when faced with a recurrence scare. An effective plan will minimize unnecessary emotional trauma and help you do the right thing.

First, look at what has triggered the scare, and ask yourself whether it is at all possible that you really do have a recurrence of your cancer. If logic tells you that your problem is not related to a recurrence, you can deal with it as you would with any other non-cancer-related problem.

If, through logical or illogical thought, you have worries or anxieties about recurrence, you need a trusted expert to tell you whether the concern is real and, if so, what must be done. In a good doctor-patient relationship, you can tell your doctor, "I know I'm fine, but I need you to tell me so." This expert is your regular doctor, either your internist, family practitioner, or oncologist.

If you are having pain that needs attention or are getting worse very quickly, call your doctor immediately. Otherwise, call your doctor's office during office hours and explain that you have a symptom that is concerning you and that you need to be seen as soon as possible.

If your doctor agrees that there is reason for concern about recurrence, be sure to do the right thing: get more information about the problem. Proceed with whatever evaluations or tests are needed. If you are advised to have a biopsy, proceed. If you do not feel comfortable with this advice, get a second opinion as soon as possible. Delaying a biopsy will not make the problem go away; it may only lessen your treatment options and lessen the chance for controlling or curing a recurrence or a noncancerous problem.

Remember that whether or not you have a recurrence is already determined at the time you notice a problem. Thinking or fearing that you might have a recurrence does not create a recurrence.

Denying that you might have a recurrence does not prevent it. You do not have a choice about whether your current symptom is due to cancer. You *do* have a choice about whether you get it evaluated. Do not waste time or energy worrying about how much you are worried or afraid. Do not try to figure out whether you are too hypochondriacal or too alarmist. When there is concern about recurrence, you can expect to have some emotions. Reassure yourself that you have a plan of action and that you are doing the right thing.

You owe it to yourself to be evaluated as soon as possible. You deserve to minimize the physical and emotional impact of any problem through early evaluation.

As you go through the motions of getting your problem evaluated, remind yourself that

- not every cough or lump is a sign of cancer
- you owe it to yourself and those people who care about you to get evaluated at the earliest opportunity, which will influence the impact of the findings
- even if it is recurrence, you can be treated again

Recurrence is not a death sentence.

For many people, it helps to imagine receiving good test results. Training yourself to stop bad-outcome scenarios in their tracks will not change the outcome, but it will definitely change the experience you have waiting for tests and evaluations to be completed. If things do not turn out well and your greatest fear is again realized, you will deal with your recurrence then. If everything turns out okay, as many times it does, you will have saved yourself much anxiety and disruption.

It helps some people to imagine bad test results and then plan how they will handle bad news, practically and emotionally. Thinking through contingency plans for work and home in case the biopsy is positive seems to offer some people a sense of control over the anxiety of the unknown. Imagining bad results makes others feel that if they think the worst, it will not happen. This is a paradoxical way of using magical thinking for comfort, but it is effective for some people.

Do what feels best to you. You may have to try different ways of coping with fear and anxiety to find the style that works best for you.

Will My Being Optimistic and Positive Make Me Feel Worse If I Do End Up Having a Recurrence in the Future?

Being diagnosed with recurrent cancer brings a traumatic, emotional, difficult time under any circumstances. There is no way to prepare for recurrence or soften the blow if it happens. If you are like most people, thinking things will be bad before you receive the diagnosis of recurrence does not make it easier to hear the news. Nor does expecting good news worsen the blow when you find out you have cancer again. The blow may feel a little different, but you face a difficult time no matter what you expected before the diagnosis.

The recurrence scare is part of cancer survivorship. Overall, the scares far outnumber the actual recurrences. It tends to be adaptive and healthy to believe you are okay unless there is proof to the contrary, as long as you take the right steps to find out for sure.

Should I Make Plans Now in Case I Get a Recurrence?

It is very rare for a recurrence to come up totally unexpectedly and then so to incapacitate you that you have little time to make adjustments or plans. Usually there are warning signs that things may not be going well, such as a suspicious test result at your follow-up or a symptom that builds gradually. You can deal with the specifics of job, school, and child care when you have to. It will be hard for you and the people around you to feel secure in your health if you are always making contingency plans for a potential recurrence.

Important plans such as wills and long-term child care arrangements are best settled now if not already settled. These responsibilities should be met by everyone whether or not there is a cancer history.

Funeral arrangements and last letters to family and friends are common concerns of survivors. Getting these details out of the way unburdens some people and frees them to forget about their cancer. For others, these acts carry too much subconscious weight, sealing their sad fate in their minds. Do what feels right to you, and then explain it to those involved so that they can understand and support you.

What If I Seem to Be Fearful of Everything, Not Just Recurrence?

You may feel fearful about everything. Every car trip represents a potential accident, every stranger a potential robber or rapist, every sunny day a potential exposure to dangerous rays, and every playground slide or swing a potential head injury for your child.

The world is not more dangerous than it was before you had cancer; it just seems more dangerous because you got hurt. Since disaster happened once, you feel that it can happen again. You can picture doctor visits and hospitals too easily, making imaginary scenarios more real. You feel very vulnerable.

This is a normal part of recovery. With time, these fears will lessen and you will feel almost, if not quite, as safe as you did before your cancer experience. Recognize where your fears come from. For the short term avoid situations that make you anxious, as long as this behavior does not interfere with your important responsibilities or have a detrimental effect on others. Avoiding anxiety-producing situations will enable you to regain a sense of control and safety again.

If you are afraid to drive on the expressway, take alternative routes. If you feel afraid when a friend invites you to try a new sport or activity, take a rain check. If you are afraid to eat certain foods, arrange your diet accordingly. You will start doing these things when you are ready.

Sometimes it is best to just face the fear and thus eliminate it. If you go ahead and drive on the expressway, you can then say, "I did it," and banish the fear. Depending on what it is you fear, how you feel, and how you like to tackle problems, you can use your judgment to decide when to avoid something and when to tackle it. If you find you cannot function at all normally or if you have significant fearfulness that does not lessen with time, get some help dealing with it.

GETTING HELP/GIVING HELP

Do I Need to Ask for Any Help after Completion of Therapy?

Cancer survivors often benefit from assistance during cancer treatments. Even after your treatments have ended, the physical effects and emotional strain continue for a variable period of time. In effect, your body is still under treatment at a time that your physical and emotional reserves are depleted. Getting help now will conserve your reserves and allow you to focus your energy on getting well again. You will spare yourself unnecessary frustration and disappointment if you learn from others the ins and outs of recovery instead of trying to discover everything for yourself.

Asking for help is a sign of courage and control. Asking for help provides others the opportunity to feel fulfilled. Asking for help promotes everyone's recovery.

What Kind of Help Do I Need?

Depending on your circumstances, you may benefit from

- continued practical help until you are stronger—for example, with meals or carpooling
- information about your current condition, your options regarding further treatment and prevention of future medical problems, and factors that will speed your recovery both physically and emotionally
- advice about coping with the physical, emotional, social, and spiritual changes
- emotional support

Where Do I Get Help?

Talk to your family and friends. Despite how you feel, it may not be obvious to them that you need help or how they can provide it. Although your needs may be less obvious than they were when you were first diagnosed, they are no less real. If you do not make them clear, family and friends who would have wanted to help may disappear from the helping scene out of ignorance. Asking for help when you need it will speed your recovery, which will benefit everyone. Allowing people to help offers them an opportunity to do something fulfilling. You help others by asking for help.

Local cancer support groups are a valuable resource. Other survivors will be able to listen to and understand your feelings and concerns, and offer real advice on how best to get and stay well.

Social workers, counselors, clergy, and psychologists can spare you unnecessary or prolonged periods of grief, depression, and anxiety by helping you define the problems and outline healthy solutions. There are some definite advantages for everyone if you work with a professional who is not personally involved in your home or family. The distance allows him or her to see and advise in areas that are too sensitive for family or friends.

Other woefully underutilized resources are the local and national hotlines, information clearinghouses, and support groups. They all provide information and support. When they cannot answer your question or need themselves, they can direct you to the resource that can. Get a listing of support services by calling your local office of the American Cancer Society, your local hospital's social work department, or the National Cancer Institute's Cancer Information Service (1-800-4CANCER). Check your telephone directory for other services under "Cancer."

How Can I Ask for Help Now, after Treatment, When I Asked for So Much during Treatment?

You may feel that it was acceptable to ask for help, support, and attention during cancer treatment but that now you should be taking care of your own needs. On the contrary, physically and emotionally you are still experiencing the effects of treatment. In many ways you bear the brunt of the experience after treatment is completed.

Cancer treatment and recovery must be considered one long process toward health. The cancer treatment was the dramatic part of the process to get you well again. Your body still has to recover physically from the cancer and the treatments. Your emotions and spirit still have to recover from the trauma and changes. The dramatic part of making a clay statue is the painstaking molding and carving. The passive last step of heating the statue in the kiln is critical in creating a lasting artwork. Making the batter and baking the cake take the most time, but icing the cake transforms it from a food to a celebration.

Physical and emotional recovery after cancer treatment is a demanding, energy-consuming process. An analogy is the case of mountain climbers who, after reaching the summit, expend great care and energy in descending; without this expediture of effort their successful ascent might be followed by disaster. Your recovery after treatment is part of your path to wellness that began with treatment.

After you complete your cancer treatment, you deserve help and support during recovery at least as much as you did during treatment.

What If I Feel the Urge to Help Other Cancer Survivors?

Helping someone else

- makes you feel that something good is coming out of your experience
- is one way to give back for the help you received
- gives you a sense of control over cancer
- allows you to save someone else a few of the hardships you may have experienced

When Can I Start Giving Back for the Help I Received?

In order to maximize your own recovery, you should wait a year or so before you formally become involved in a program to help other cancer survivors.

Many situations will arise where you are called on for advice or support by newly diagnosed patients or families of a cancer patient. You may feel obligated to help because

- people helped you when you were sick
- you empathize with the distress of a newly diagnosed patient
- you do not want the caller to feel abandoned

Whether or not you make yourself available and how deeply you become involved must be decided on a day-by-day and case-by-case basis. Factors to consider include

- how comfortable you feel with your own situation
- how many physical or emotional problems of your own you are dealing with
- how many people are calling on you
- how many other responsibilities you have
- how tired you are
- how much time you have
- how great the needs of the person requesting help are
- how you feel after you help others

Wait a few weeks or months to help others if, right now, talking to others leaves you exhausted, fearful, or distraught and unable to sleep. You must balance your physical and emotional needs against the needs of your family and the needs of the person requesting help. For a while you have to protect yourself from too much avoidable emotional stress. Other people may not recognize that you have depleted reserves, that you are still dealing with your own issues, or that helping others is especially draining if you do not have much distance from your own cancer experience.

Dealing with someone else's cancer is a complicated task. For everyone's sake, bear in mind that you are not a mental health professional and should not burden yourself with a situation better handled by someone with training. It is possible that you are still dealing with unresolved issues related to your own cancer that could be reopened by the relationship with a newly diagnosed patient. You need to be aware of your own stage of emotional recovery in order to best serve someone else.

The best way you can help everyone is to take care of yourself. There will be plenty of opportunities to help others when the time is right for you.

Won't I Feel Guilty If I Don't Help Someone Else?

Your top priority at this time is to recover as safely and quickly as possible. If someone else's needs are too great for you to handle now, letting someone else take care of the person's needs is the best decision you can make for everyone's sake. You can help others by referring them to services and people who are in a position to help.

STRAINED RELATIONSHIPS

What If There Is More Stress at Home since My Treatments Ended?

Transitions, whether good or bad, bring stress. A change in job, marriage status, number of children in the home, living arrangements, or stage of schooling brings stress. Completing treatment marks a significant transition. There are decisions and adjustments to make and uncertainties to face. Everyone's role and responsibilities may change. The routine that was established during the course of treatment may now be altered.

Since aggressive treatment is now over, repressed emotions may come to the surface. For the first time, family members may express anger, frustration, fear, and depression. They would not allow themselves to feel pessimistic, anxious, or depressed while you were sick, because they felt they had to be "up" for everyone's sake. Now that you are out of danger, they feel they can "let down" and allow all the pent-up feelings to come out.

Everyone is tired after your ordeal. When people are tired, they are less patient, less rational, less understanding.

If Members of My Family Seem Overly Concerned about Their Own Health, What Should I Do?

A family member with a possible medical problem should be encouraged to undergo evaluation by a trusted doctor as soon as possible. Remind him or her that an objective professional evaluation is in everyone's best interest whether or not a significant problem exists. They will either get attention to a problem when it is most treatable or be reassured that no significant problem exists.

If family members seem too concerned about their diet, environmental exposures, or levels of stress, validate their health concerns as a normal aftereffect of living with cancer and its treatment. Family members' attention to their lifestyle is one way for them to regain a sense of control over their health.

How Do I Deal with Other People?

You have to take the lead in teaching family, friends, and acquaintances how best to help you and deal with you. Be direct. Tell people,

- "I appreciate your asking how I'm doing" or "It would make it easier if you didn't ask me how I'm doing all the time, and let me tell you when something is happening, or when I feel like talking."
- "I still need help doing things and appreciate your willingness to continue to help me" or "I feel that I can do things myself now, and I feel better when you encourage me to do things myself."
- "It helps me to talk about my cancer experience and the issues with which I'm now dealing" or "It helps me *not* to talk about my cancer experience and to try to focus on other things."
- "I need space and quiet time" or "I need company and activities."

What helps you or hurts you may change from day to day, or even hour to hour. Sometimes you may not be sure what you want or need. Let your friends and family know that you appreciate their concern and recognize that it is sometimes hard to know how to relate.

SUPPORT GROUPS

Do I Need to Participate in a Support Group?

Having completed treatment, you may think, "Why would I need a support group now?" After a diagnosis of cancer, the initial challenge is to get through treatment. The longer-term challenge is to find a place for your cancer history in your life so that it enhances, not detracts from, the rest of your life.

If you are having any concerns, anxieties, worries, fears, or depression after you complete your treatments, a support group might be an excellent place for working through these normal negative feelings as efficiently and painlessly as possible.

If you feel very healthy, physically and emotionally, and sense that your life is getting back to normal easily, you probably do not need a support group. It might be nice to go to give advice to others who are having a more difficult time than you.

If you are feeling lonely, one of the best remedies is a good support group. In general, people who attend a support group are motivated to find healthy ways to cope. You may find the advice of other survivors not only practical but also inspirational. Sharing with other cancer survivors helps dissipate loneliness and the sense of alienation that often accompanies surviving. Listening to other people who have faced and overcome some of the problems you are facing will help diminish any "Why me?" or "Nobody understands" feelings.

Won't It Be Depressing or Scary to Be with Other Cancer Patients?

All support groups are different. Even the same support group is different at each meeting, depending on the individuals who attend that day and the topics discussed. The person in charge of the meeting, the facilitator, can make a major difference in the flow and tone of the meetings.

At many support groups, you cannot tell the patients from the friends and family members by how they look. There is often lots of laughter and joking, as well as exchange of practical information and genuine support. Try attending a support group for two or three sessions before you decide whether it will be helpful for you.

Do Support Groups Work?

Many well-documented scientific studies show a correlation between support group attendance and improved quality of life. A 1989 study of women with metastatic breast cancer showed a significant improvement in survival time in those who received weekly supportive group therapy. If the group is good, and you feel comfortable in it, you will doubtless enjoy improved quality of life and, possibly, length of life.

How Do I Find Out about the Local Support Groups?

To find out more about the support groups in your area, call

- your local hospital's social work department
- the local office of the American Cancer Society
- the Cancer Information Service (1-800-4CANCER)

THE MIND–BODY CONNECTION

Is There a Connection between the Mind and the Body?

Absolutely. Picture in your mind's eye the following: You are picking up a firm, bright yellow lemon. Then, you slice it in half, and a few squirts of juice hit your face, and your fingertips get soaked. Bring the lemon up to your nose, and take a whiff. Lick the cut surface of the lemon. Take a bite.

If you noticed an increased flow of saliva in your mouth as you read the description, you have observed how the mind can affect the body. Just thinking about the lemon caused measurable changes in your body. If you had no response, read the paragraph more slowly, concentrating on each phrase, pausing between phrases, really trying to imagine yourself tasting the lemon.

The mind can affect the body, and the body can affect the mind. Pain, fatigue, medications, and hormonal imbalances can affect mood, concentration, and other functions of the mind.

A new field of science, psychoneuroimmunology, is investigating the relationship between the mind and the body. Research is starting to reveal some of the mechanisms by which the mind interacts with the body. It is hoped that we will soon be able to harness and amplify the beneficial healing powers of the mind.

Given that the mind and the body are connected, several questions arise: How much *does* the mind affect the body? How much *can* the mind affect the body? Does your mind cause you to develop cancer? Can your mind heal cancer or prevent recurrence?

Are There Different Types of Stress?

Negative stress is stress that makes you feel bad or overtaxes you. Divorce, financial worries, and job insecurity are examples of negative emotional stresses. Starvation and frequent marathon running are examples of negative physical stresses.

Positive stress is stress that energizes you. Projects and promotions are examples of positive emotional stresses. Daily aerobic exercise and a low-fat diet when you need to lose weight are examples of positive physical stresses.

Whether something is a positive or a negative stress for you depends on how you respond to it. What is energizing and fun for one person may be fatiguing and depressing for you.

What Is the Relationship between Stress and Control of My Cancer?

Stress is only one factor that affects health. There are unsubstantiated claims that too much negative stress or poorly handled positive stress can affect your immune system in an adverse way. It is suggested that a depressed immune system cannot fight infections or control cancer cells as well as a healthy immune system.

Solid data correlating stress and cancer in humans are lacking. There are no scientific data to support the notion that stress is a cause of cancer or a cause of recurrence. Anecdotes are not scientific evidence.

Stress only affects your health; it does not control your health.

Could My Mind Have Caused My Cancer?

Your mind affects your health, often in profound ways, but it does not control your health. Wishing yourself to get sick, either consciously or subconsciously, will not cause you to develop cancer. Having cancer does not mean that you, either consciously or subconsciously, wanted to get cancer. Many factors within and beyond your control determined that you developed cancer and when you developed it.

Your mind affects your health by playing a role in your choice of diet, use of alcohol or other harmful substances, participation in an exercise program, and choice of job or living arrangements. These factors are known to influence your risk of developing cancer.

Your mind affects how you interface with your life. If you react to difficulties with genuine calm and hope, your body's reaction will be very different from what it would be if you reacted with anxiety or bottled-up anger. There is scientific evidence for the health benefits of joy, laughter, love, and relaxation in your life. Unpleasant stress, chronic anger or frustration, and major loss are harmful to your health.

Your overall happiness and your ability to deal with stress are only two factors that affect your health. A well-balanced life does not make you immune to cancer. If you cope poorly with difficult life circumstances, you are not guaranteed a short life. If the mind controlled health, happy people would never die from cancer. Depressed, rejected, abandoned, or grief-stricken people who had difficulty coping would all die prematurely of heart attacks or cancer. But we all know people who were genuinely happy before they developed cancer, and many miserable people who lived to a ripe old age.

Scientific studies that have tried to look at the relationship between the development of cancer and a person's state of mind, or a person's life stresses, such as losing a spouse or becoming unemployed, have given conflicting results. Even the studies that support the association between stress and cancer provide no scientific data to show that stress causes cancer or its recurrence.

Your mind affects your health but does not control it.

What If I Am Worried That the Way I Deal with Stress Caused My Cancer or Can Cause My Cancer to Recur?

You can easily lose sight of the fact that there is no scientific evidence that stress causes cancer. You may be bombarded by urgings from friends and family to control the stress in your life because you have had cancer. Even casual comments take their toll: "I told you that you were working too hard." "You can't afford to get all wrapped up in everyone's problems any more."

The idea that you caused your cancer and can control your future health is reinforced by many popular self-help books. They suggest that you developed cancer because of repressed hostility, because you spent your life taking care of others' needs instead of your own, or because you did not love yourself enough.

Dr. Bernie Siegel, in his best-selling book *Love, Medicine, and Miracles,* makes broad statements based on anecdotes and theory, not on fact. He states that 15–20 percent of all patients unconsciously, or even consciously, wish to die. He later states that the onset and course of disease are strongly linked to a person's ability and willingness to cope with stress.

The aim of such self-help books is not to make you feel guilty about having gotten cancer but to make you feel empowered. If your mind could cause your cancer, changes in how you think, feel, and live will keep you from having cancer again. Siegel's words of empowerment excite readers by claiming that potentially all patients can learn to heal themselves and stay well, that the course of your disease is strongly linked to your ability and willingness to cope with stress, and that if you can believe that you will get well, you have laid the foundation for your cure. He asserts that your attitude toward yourself is the single most important factor in healing or staying well and that your decisions concerning such things as eating, sleeping, smoking, exercising, and wearing seat belts control about 90 percent of the factors that determine your state of health. Not one of these assertions is based on scientific fact. Siegel's books are best-sellers because people want to have control over their health and their lives. He offers you this sense of control.

Love, Medicine, and Miracles presents some wonderful points, such as the importance of working as a team with your doctor and trusting your doctor, the value of support groups, and the limitations of statistics. It offers healthy philosophies, such as the idea that there is always hope, that there is no such thing as false hope, and that the key to a full life is aiming for personal peace and peace with those around you.

Unfortunately, interlaced with his helpful messages is the dangerous theme that you are responsible for your illness, for getting well and staying well. Dealing with cancer is difficult enough without the added burden of misplaced guilt. Trying to avoid stress or trying to control your response to unavoidable changes and losses can be extremely stressful and unrealistic.

Life is full of good and bad stresses. To be human is to be involved with others, and to feel life's pain and sorrow. Unless you are an unfeeling zombie, living well will include times of grief and frustration. The only way for you to avoid life's stresses is to hide from the world. This would mean hiding from all of life's joys, too. The whole reason for surviving cancer is to live your life, not to hide from it.

After surviving cancer, you should indeed try to change circumstances that cause unpleasant stress, to improve relationships, and to accept and love yourself. These changes will enhance your quality of life and help you get and stay well.

At the same time, though, remember that you cannot control the world around you. You are not doomed to recurrence if you lose your job, or get in an argument with your child, or grieve over the loss of a loved one. Your body can handle normal life events, especially if you are honest with yourself and share your feelings. Getting adequate rest and eating well are two concrete ways of helping your body deal with stress. Minimize the detrimental effects of stress by learning to decrease negative stress, handle unavoidable stress, and turn negative stress into positive stress. Find a balance between what is known scientifically about the mind–body connection and your own beliefs.

What Are Negative Thoughts?

Negative thoughts are thoughts about things not going well. "I'm going to have a recurrence." "My energy is never going to get better." Some people call them "dark thoughts." When they are subconscious, you have them before you realize that you are having them. When they are conscious, you actively construct bad thoughts about your cancer, your situation, your health, your death. Negative thoughts are unpleasant. They make you feel depressed, anxious, afraid, or angry.

What If I Have Negative Thoughts?

Negative thoughts provide one of the ways that your subconscious works out problems or expresses sources of fear, anxiety, anger, or depression.

If I Have Negative Thoughts, Does That Mean That Deep Inside I Believe That I Will Do Poorly?

Negative thoughts reflect what you fear. Most cancer survivors have negative thoughts at some time or other. Even the most optimistic, secure, faithful cancer survivor has occasional negative thoughts when he or she is scheduled for a checkup or being evaluated for a new symptom. Frequent or obsessive negative thoughts can indicate a more serious medical or emotional problem that requires attention.

The important question is not whether you have negative thoughts but what you do with them.

Negative thoughts reveal your fears and concerns, not your beliefs.

What Is the Effect of My Negative Thoughts on My Body?

Negative thoughts can be disruptive, making you feel anxious, hopeless, or depressed. The effect of negative thoughts depends on your response to them. If you dismiss them as normal and insignificant, they will have little impact on your health. If you give them a lot of emphasis, the resulting emotions can cause physiological and behavioral changes that are not conducive to good health.

Negative thoughts do not cause cancer. If they did, everyone would have recurrences.

What Should I Do If I Have Occasional Negative Thoughts?

Define your negative thought and see whether you can identify what triggered it. If it is something obvious like going for a checkup, recognize the source of the negative thought and retrain yourself to dissolve these negative thoughts. (See the section on checkup anxiety, pp. 236–38.)

If you cannot identify the cause, define the negative thought and its meaning more closely and try again to figure out the cause.

Practice interrupting negative thoughts. Direct your thoughts to healthy, optimistic alternatives. Diminish the anxiety associated with negative thoughts through self-hypnosis or relaxation techniques.

Reassure yourself that occasional negative thoughts are a normal part of the survivorship territory and can be disempowered.

Reassure yourself that occasional negative thoughts do not reflect badly on your optimism about yourself. Remind yourself that negative thoughts do not cause cancer or other illness.

What Are Magical Thinking and Superstition?

Magical thinking is believing that your thoughts can cause changes or events in the real world when it is impossible for them to do so. It is magical thinking when you believe that it rained on your outdoor wedding because the week before the big day you thought, "It is going to rain on my wedding day." It is magical thinking if you believe that by thinking, "I am going to have a recurrence," you will cause a recurrence.

Superstition, in contrast to magical thinking, is a custom or act believed to cause a desired event or to prevent an undesired one. Children utilize superstition often—for example, when they close the curtains to keep out the witches. Since ancient times, cultures have passed on superstitions, such as that of Italian and Jewish families that tie a red ribbon on a new baby's crib to ward off the evil spirits. You are repeating one when you cross two fingers of one hand to bring someone good luck (crossing two fingers of each hand supposedly brings bad luck). People engage in personalized superstitious customs, such as when a wife utters the same words before every single departure of her husband, "Drive carefully; I'll see you later," fearing that misfortune will result if she does not.

Superstition is also the irrational belief that something or some circumstance portends something bad. That superstition persists today is obvious when you see hospitals and hotels without a thirteenth floor (the twelfth floor is followed by the fourteenth), people throwing salt over their left shoulder, or going out of their way not to walk under a ladder or step on a crack.

You may have developed a repertoire of personal superstitions to help you cope with the uncertainties of life. You may take a special route or wear a designated outfit to every one of your checkups, if it was the route you took or outfit you wore the day your remission was announced.

Are Magical Thinking and Superstitious Thinking Normal?

Magical thinking is left over from childhood, when normal individuals believe that their thoughts can cause some of the changes in their world that they do not understand, or can protect them from the things they fear. Children believe that thinking that there will be a snowstorm can bring about the snow holiday, or that their mom got cancer because, in a moment of anger before she got sick, they thought, "I wish she would die."

As we grow older, we use less and less magical thinking, but we all engage in magical thinking to some degree, believing that our thoughts can help bring about good things, ward off bad, and explain events. Adults allay their fear of flying by telling themselves that the mission is too important for the jet to crash. Frightened patients promise to quit smoking, hoping or believing that eleventh-hour promises will help the biopsy turn out benign. Survivors of car crashes tell themselves that they should not have gone out just because of a sale on their favorite shoes and that this is why they were in an accident.

As we gain understanding of or control over such phenomena as the weather, old superstitions often die. However, many superstitions persist, even in the face of scientific evidence to the contrary. People adopt cultural and family superstitions as part of their identity, to reinforce their sense of belonging, just as they follow current hairstyles or dress codes. In addition, superstitions afford them an accepted way to gain a sense of control over their world.

Are Magical Thinking and Superstition Healthy?

Magical thinking persists into adulthood and superstition into the modern era because of their ability to offer comfort and a sense of control over things that are beyond human control.

The belief that you will never be in an accident, because you are charmed, provides comfort beyond that offered by wearing seat belts and driving defensively. The belief that your thinking, "I am going to see my daughter graduate from school" or "I am going to finish this project," will make it so relieves understandable but unproductive anxiety about dying before important times.

Are Magical Thinking or Superstition Ever Harmful?

Magical thinking and superstition are harmful when they

- keep you from doing the right thing
- cause strained relationships
- cause additional fear or anxiety
- make you feel depressed
- keep you from functioning normally

One woman had been told as a child that she would never get hurt in a car. Believing that she was charmed, as she grew up, she never wore a seat belt. Magical thinking protected her from anxiety about the dangers of driving, but prevented her from taking proper precautions. Another woman believed that her cancer was caused by the routine vaccination she had received prior to her diagnosis, and so she refused any further vaccinations. Magical thinking, which offered her the comfort of an answer to the "Why me?" question, kept her from getting important vaccinations.

The belief that your occasional thoughts of recurrence will cause you to have cancer again magnifies your normal fear of recurrence and can paralyze you if not recognized. If you should have a recurrence, this irrational belief would add an unnecessary burden of guilt during an already stressful time.

Superstitions that prevent you from doing the right thing are dangerous. One man with heart and lung disease developed appendicitis, but refused to have the necessary surgery, because it was the thirteenth day of the month. His routine appendicitis developed into a ruptured appendix with peritonitis, and he died.

Superstitions that cause or exacerbate fear, anxiety, or hopelessness are harmful. If every episode of car trouble or leaf falling off a houseplant portends your imminent death, you will waste enormous energy trying to repress or relieve the anxiety inflamed by superstitious thinking.

Let magical thinking and superstitions bring you comfort. Do not let them keep you from doing the right thing, or adding unnecessary stress, strain, anxiety, or guilt.

DEALING WITH THE FUTURE

What If I Have Trouble Thinking about My Future or Picturing Good Things in My Future?

Cancer made your future seem less certain. Soon after treatment is completed, you may feel that you are safe only for a day, a week, a month, or a few months.

Picturing the future may elicit enormous anxiety, anger, or sadness because you fear that you may not get to experience it. You can experience anticipatory grief when picturing the future because projecting the future is a setup for allowing a glimpse of all possible future outcomes, including the fearsome one of illness and death. This occurs even if your prognosis is good and you are picturing happy events, such as a graduation, marriage, or the birth of a child.

What If I Have Trouble Planning for the Future?

Planning for the future means having confidence that the plans will come to fruition. You lost a lot when you got cancer. You feel vulnerable. You want to protect yourself from avoidable loss and pain. If, on any level, you are insecure about your future, you will feel anxious when you start to make plans, because you do not want to lose any more.

Sometimes a component of magical thinking makes it difficult for you to make plans. You may feel that if you make plans, you are setting yourself up for a problem that will sabotage the plans. "If I don't make plans, there won't be any plans to get ruined. If there are no plans to ruin, I won't get cancer."

How Can I Start to Re-create My Future?

Figure out how much time you feel safe thinking about and stick to that time frame. If you feel fairly confident that you will be at least as healthy tomorrow as you are today, make plans to do something tomorrow—have lunch with someone, visit a park, or talk to a friend on the phone. When tomorrow comes, carry out your plans. As you feel better and get involved with non-cancer-related activities, you will feel safer about greater periods of your future. It takes time without medical problems to help you feel safe about the future.

Remember that people who have never had cancer usually focus most of their energies on the present and on the immediate future, and only occasionally on the distant future. Parents with very small children spend little time picturing their children as teenagers or young adults concerned about career and family life. Active, middle-aged people spend little time wondering or worrying about what event or illness will precipitate their death. Even very elderly people who are active and involved in the world around them focus on the immediate future.

When you catch yourself imagining bad outcomes to plans for the future, consciously adjust the picture in your mind to a good outcome. If you cannot do this, turn it off. You are not ready to deal with the future. Counseling may help you to sort out what fears are making it difficult for you to picture the future and to learn how to tame those fears.

Planning for the future does not control the future. It helps you live today and tomorrow. Planning to watch a special show on television or visit with a friend allows you the pleasure of anticipation and gives you a little foothold on the future. If it does not come to pass, little is lost.

Many survivors help diminish their anxiety about the future by consciously making plans. One woman buys a new outfit at end-of-the-season sales. She knows that she will not be able to wear it this year, but the purchase is her statement to herself that she plans to be around next year to wear it. One man renews his magazine subscriptions for three years at a time as his way of demonstrating his desire and will to be here. Instead of allowing his anxiety about his future to control him, he challenges his fear, giving him some sense of control.

Making plans for the future, even if the future is merely a few hours from now, is a way to validate and energize your present. Living in the present requires thoughts and actions that take you into the future.

"WHY ME?"

What If I Am Asking "Why Me?" Now?

Interestingly, some people ask "Why me?" for the first time after treatment is completed. Shock, confusion, and preoccupation with the treatments may have kept you from asking this philosophical question until you tried to reintegrate yourself into the healthy world. The contrast between how other people look and feel and how you look and feel highlights just how much you have suffered and lost.

Why Me?

This is an age-old question that touches on your beliefs about the meaning of life and about God. The human condition is one that includes pain, loss, and death. There is no escaping the human condition. Use the question "Why me?" as a stimulus to explore your beliefs. Books, clergy, friends, and family can help you work toward an acceptable answer, or toward peace with no answer.

From a cold, practical point of view, unless the chance of your developing your type of cancer was zero before your diagnosis, your developing cancer was consistent with the probability. For example, if you had a 1-in-1,000 chance of getting leukemia, developing leukemia would be in keeping with the probability.

From a more philosophical or existential view, the corollary question "Why not me?" may induce you to let the "Why me?" question rest.

If understanding the human condition does not quell your anger, disappointment, envy, confusion, or depression associated with seeing other people go along their apparently merry way while you struggle with recovery from cancer treatment, or if "Why me?" continues to affect your thoughts and feelings, seek assistance from clergy or counselors. Getting stuck in "Why me?" will trap you in your diagnosis. Finding acceptable answers or alternative, answerable questions will liberate you to move forward.

Find peace with the "Why me?" question so that you can move on to a more practical one: "What can I do about my situation now?"

5

Insights and Handles to Help
You Get to Your New Life

Many millions of people have recovered from cancer. The experience of these veterans provides insights and handles for helping you through the transition to your new life after cancer. There is no way to eliminate all the emotions, discomforts, inconveniences, worries, strains, and uncertainties. However, you can learn ways to cope with the difficulties of recovery and living with a cancer history. You can learn tricks and philosophies that will make the hard times easier.

Elaborate investigation and analysis of a problem serve a purpose. But at times a simple phrase helps more than all the sophisticated, caring discussion in the world. You can spend hours discussing the fear of recurrence, but sometimes saying, "Recurrence is not a death sentence," is all you want or need. After investigation and analysis, a simple phrase can help you recapture all the derived insights and benefits at a later time, without going through the tedious process again. You can learn about the family dynamics when one member is sick, but at times you are best served by the simple statement "Cancer is a family affair."

Handles are aids for moving from one place to another. Their usefulness depends as much on the person using them and the place where the person is going as on the handle itself. Some handles may become your mantras of self-help, providing dependable comfort and inspiration whenever you feel the need. You may find other handles worthless to you. Specific handles may be helpful to you only under certain circumstances or at different times in your life. If the handles help you, use them. If they do not, look for other handles that do. The following are offered to make your transition to your new life as safe and smooth as possible.

The roller coaster of cancer.

Having cancer and undergoing cancer treatments are often compared to being on a roller coaster: good days and bad days, easy days and rough days, peaceful days and stressful days, hopeful days and disappointing days, comfortable days and uncomfortable days. The ride does not stop with your last treatment. Be prepared for posttreatment medical problems and emotional upsets.

Checkups, tests, and cancer- and treatment-related problems cause fluctuating anxiety, frustration, depression, and disappointment. As time goes on and your cancer history recedes farther into your past, the ups and downs will smooth out.

The tools you have acquired through your cancer experience will help you deal with the non-cancer-related trials of life in such a way that you can end up with a smoother ride after cancer than before.

Expect strong emotions and reactions.

Your reactions and emotions after finishing treatment are real, no matter how extreme. The completion of treatment marks a major transition, in which you and your family again face the seriousness of your situation. Strong emotions are also expected after checkups, at holidays and anniversaries, and when potential and real problems occur. Overall, strong emotions will lessen with time. Strong emotions show that you are thoughtful and connected to the world around you. You would have to be an unthinking, unfeeling zombie to get past posttreatment milestones without experiencing any emotions.

What emotions you have is less important than what you do with them.

Strong emotions are not a problem unless they keep you from doing the right things. They are your body's communication system for letting you know how you are doing and what you need to work on. Instead of worrying about the fact that you are so fearful, spend your energy exploring the source of your fears and ways to tame them. If you are angry, discover the source of your anger and find ways to dissipate or resolve your anger.

No matter what you are feeling, do the right thing.

A fireman is a professional who learns to brave flames and save burning victims, no matter what fear of flames or revulsion at burning flesh he or she feels. You can learn how to be a professional survivor, doing the right thing to prevent and stave off problems, no matter what you are feeling. Do the right thing for your overall health, no matter how you look or feel doing it. If you cannot, because of fear, emotions, or uncertainty about what the right thing is, get help.

Recovery after cancer is a family affair.

The cancer experience happened to you and everyone around you. Recovery, too, is a family affair. Despite the relief that your treatment is over, everyone has heightened anxiety and worry. Roles change, feelings are unleashed, and new problems surface. You will help yourself by being tuned in to those around you. Illness and recovery do not release you from the need to be sensitive to those around you, as much as you can.

Focus on what you can do to help your recovery and maintain your renewed health.

There are many things you can do to facilitate your recovery and preserve your renewed health. Instead of worrying about bad things that could happen or things you cannot control, focus on realistic ways to strengthen your physical, emotional, and spiritual health. Efforts toward progress, no matter how small, are life enhancing.

Worrying about your past or your future poisons your present.
Regretting or worrying about what you did, what you did not do, and what you could have done is a waste of time, energy, and emotion. You can never change the past. If you find yourself ruminating on the past, train yourself to focus on what you can do now to improve your health and enrich your life emotionally and spiritually.

Worrying about your future is also a waste of time, energy, and emotion. You may be worrying about a problem that will never materialize, in which case a nonexistent problem is causing you distress. Worrying now will not help you get through a situation that does develop in the future; it just prolongs and deepens the pain caused by the problem. You do not have to be free of all anxiety about your future before you can enjoy your present. Whenever you feel that you are living in a never-never land of "wait and see," try to think of yourself as surviving in the land of "live and see."

Cancer victims and cancer survivors are people in the same situation with a different frame of mind.
Focus on what you still have and what you have gained, not on what you have lost. Focus on what you can do, not on what you cannot do. Two people in the same situation can experience their lives completely differently, depending on how they focus. How you experience your life depends on your state of mind.

Control is an illusion.
Having cancer and undergoing cancer treatment make you painfully aware of how little control you have over important things in your life. Checkups, posttreatment medical problems, and social problems can be unwelcome reminders of your vulnerability. Remember that complete control is an illusion. Your cancer did not create a loss of control; it revealed the lack of control. If anything, the tools and strengths that you can gain through your cancer experience will allow you to exercise more control over your life after cancer.

Pursue things that help; avoid things that do not.
You can shape your environment by choosing the tools you use to cope. The more tools you have, the more flexibility you will have for coping well with different situations. Support groups, helping others, reading, long discussions, private time, and exercise will be helpful or harmful depending on the circumstances and your feelings at the moment. Be willing to try varied activities and approaches over and over in order to find what works best for you at the time.

Learn to control your reaction to bad thoughts or feelings.
Isolated thoughts do not cause cancer recurrence. Everyone has unpleasant or pessimistic thoughts. Recognize these thoughts, accept them as normal phenomena, and then shift to more constructive, optimistic thoughts. You cannot always stop bad thoughts, but you can control your reaction to them. If you are troubled by frequent, persistent negative thoughts, counseling will help you sort out the source of these thoughts, find healthy ways to react, and thus gain control over them.

Grieve your new losses.
Many people feel that there is nothing left to lose after treatment. However, because of priorities during treatment, many things were nonissues until treatment was completed. Ongoing or new problems can cause raw losses. The human response to loss is grief, and there is no way to bypass the painful grieving process. Only after you have adequately grieved all the big and little losses will you feel more comfortable and content in your new normal condition.

Laugh every day.
Genuine laughter offers physical and psychological benefits in a most pleasurable way. It gives you a brief break from problems and seriousness, relieves tension between you and others, and lightens otherwise oppressive situations. Practice looking for humor all around you. Develop a ready set of quips for crises.

Set realistic goals and nourish inspiring dreams.
Working toward goals and dreams gives direction, meaning, fuel, and dignity to your present, no matter how great or mundane the

goal or how lofty the dream. Accomplishing your goals will do much to heal insecurity born of physical and emotional losses and changes. Set short-term goals for the hour or day, as well as longer-term, bigger goals. Revise your goals if they are frustratingly out of reach or not challenging enough.

Nourish dreams that comfort and energize you. Remember, dreams are the stuff of life.

Comparisons to your old self or to others are counterproductive.

Train yourself to avoid comparing your current situation or self to your precancer one. Avoid comparing yourself to people who are not dealing with cancer and to others who are. It is nourishing to be inspired by someone else's achievements but defeating to compare.

Look toward building a new you as opposed to re-creating the old you.

Trying to recapture the you before cancer is a goal destined for failure or at least major frustration. Your body, emotions, and perspective are different. Physically, think of yourself as building up to a new you, not back to your old self. Recognize your limits and handicaps so that you can work on overcoming the ones that can be overcome and accepting the ones that are unalterable. Emotionally, make your survival such a strengthening force that, after time for adequate healing, you feel unstoppable.

Focus on the good things that have come from your cancer experience.

Make a long list of the good things that have come from your cancer experience. Have them ready in your mind or, better yet, on a piece of paper kept in your wallet. At moments when you feel discouraged, angry, frustrated, or depressed, review your list. Although your situation may not change, thinking positively will help you see and feel it differently.

What does not kill you makes you strong.

Nietzsche's words can apply to you. Like survivors of wars or serious accidents, you have faced a challenge greater than any that many people ever face in their lifetime. And you survived. Take pride and gather inner strength from the fact of your survival. If you can survive cancer, you can survive other challenges.

During the immediate recovery phase, when you are still experiencing physical problems and changes and when you face a host of transitional stresses, you may feel that the experience has left you weaker and more vulnerable, not stronger. What does not kill you makes you strong *in the long run*. Immediately following a fight or challenge the victor is tired and weak. In the long run the victor is stronger.

Break up life's challenges into manageable pieces.
Every task, no matter how big, is composed of smaller, more easily managed parts. Learn how much you can handle, physically and emotionally, and then approach your life by focusing on the manageable. If you worry about how you are going to make it to your next checkup three months hence, just think about getting through the month, or week, or day. Ask yourself to handle what you know you can handle.

You do not have to be completely recovered to be really living or to feel happy.
You do not have to be free of all physical or emotional reminders of your cancer before you can get on with your real life. All of your sensations and experiences are real. Waiting for everything to be back to normal before you see yourself as really living is a waste of precious time. There is no time like the present.

Acceptance is like a wave.
Some of the changes in your life may happen quickly, over seconds, days, weeks, or months. Acceptance of the changes and their consequences, however, takes longer. You can know you have cancer and take all the right steps to treat your cancer for a long time before you totally accept your illness. Acceptance is a complicated process with many levels, something that happens gradually over days, weeks, months, and years. It is like a wave, coming in and out over time, slowly making progress on the reef of denial, in contrast to a light switch, which with one flick illuminates the stark reality.

Pamper yourself.

Reward yourself. You have been through a lot. You deserve it. Doing something special for yourself is not taking advantage of your situation or making cancer therapy more attractive. It validates self-worth and demonstrates freedom.

Knowledge is power.

Knowledge, no matter how devastating, helps you. Knowledge diminishes your anxiety and fear and allows you to be your own best advocate. Having knowledge does not change the facts; it enables you to use them to your advantage.

There is nothing to fear but fear itself.

Franklin D. Roosevelt's words provide a powerful handle for cancer survivors. Fear is a normal human response that is good only when it helps you to do the right thing. Unbridled, unproductive fear is debilitating and steals otherwise good-quality life from you. Learn to tame your fears and recapture your life.

Your mind affects your health; it does not control your health.

Use your powerful mind to your advantage. Learn how to harness the self-healing and self-comforting capabilities of your mind. At the same time recognize that ultimate control of your health and your life is out of your hands.

There are always choices.

You cannot always choose your circumstances, but you can always choose how you deal with them. Even when your choices are severely limited, acting on the choices you do have is liberating.

Learning to cope with challenges gives you the strength to face them and the confidence that you can get through them.

Epilogue

It has been two and a half years since I started this book. My professional and personal exposure has brought me into contact with hundreds of people struggling to feel normal after cancer. Although I, like other cancer survivors, have faced and must continue to deal with problems, there *are* ways to avoid, diminish, or overcome these obstacles to a healthy new life.

Living with cancer and its aftereffects is an ongoing education in living in general. For me, it has been an opportunity to learn about myself, my life, my family and friends, my faith, my community, and the age-old question of the meaning of it all.

I cannot protect myself from the pain and work of facing the hills and mountains in my life's road. Losses and disappointments will hurt, no matter how much I understand the dynamics behind my feelings and no matter how much I try to prepare. The death of a friend, recurrence of cancer, or loss of a bodily function will cause painful thoughts and feelings. Fear and anxiety will try to be ever-present companions, demanding continuous efforts to keep them tamed.

However, having learned skills for dealing with life's challenges, I am now spared the additional pain and anxiety that come from being unsure whether I *can* get to the other side of the mountain, and from fear of what I will discover and have to endure. The steady stream of information, advice, love, caring, and prayers from family, friends, and health care professionals has buoyed my confidence to know that I can handle any challenge, no matter the outcome.

Your cancer experience does not end with your last treatment. Being knowledgeable about life after cancer treatment brings comfort and better medical treatment. Understanding the changes brought on by cancer treatment allows you to join the ranks of those who have survived the cancer experience and found themselves better for it.

APPENDIX I

Glossary

acupressure. A technique to treat symptoms (such as pain) or a disease (such as cancer) by which pressure is applied to special points on the body. It offers some patients symptom relief but has not been shown to be effective in treating cancer.

acute. Marked by a severe symptom or problem that develops quickly and lasts a short time (such as acute appendicitis or acute abdominal pain due to gallstones).

adenocarcinoma. A cancer that started in glandular tissue (e.g., breast, lung, thyroid, colon, pancreas).

adenoma. A noncancerous tumor composed of glandular tissue (such as breast, lung, thyroid, colon, pancreas).

adjuvant therapy. Another form of therapy in addition to the primary form; therapy given when all available tests show no evidence of cancer. Adjuvant therapy is given in hopes of killing undetectable leftover cancer cells and of decreasing the chance of a recurrence.

ADL. Activities of daily living.

alkylating agents. A class of anticancer drugs that combine with a cancer cell's DNA to prevent cell division.

allogeneic transplant. Transfer of an organ or bone marrow sample from one person to another who is not an identical twin.

alopecia. Hair loss.

alternative therapy. Treatment that is offered for the control or cure of cancer instead of conventional medical therapy, such as laetrile, herbal tonics, homeopathy, acupuncture, and metabolic therapy.

amenorrhea. Cessation of menses (menstrual periods).

analgesic. Pain medication or treatment that works in a conscious patient.

anaplastic. A cancer whose cells, under the microscope, look very immature and different from the tissue in which the cancer started. These are usually faster-growing cancers.

androgens. Male sex hormones.

anecdotal evidence. Evidence, sometimes presented to support a scientific argument, that is based on hearsay or isolated examples. Such evidence is not reliable, because it is not based on a systematic collection of data. The information obtained from it can be biased, and is not controlled to determine the cause of the claimed result.

anemia. "Low blood count"; low red blood cells or hemoglobin as a result of blood loss, blood destruction in the vessels, or impaired ability to make new blood.

angiogram. X ray of blood vessels taken after the injection of dye.

anorexia. Lack of appetite.

antibody. A protein made by the body in response to a foreign protein (such as a protein on a bacterium or cancer cell).

anticoagulant. A substance that slows or prevents blood clotting.

antiemetic. Treatment to prevent nausea or vomiting.

antigens. Substances that activate the immune system to make antibodies.

antimetabolites. A class of anticancer drugs that interfere with cancer cell metabolism.

antioxidants. Substances found in tiny amounts that serve as the body's defense against free radicals and reactive oxygen molecules (by-products of normal body function that are thought to damage normal cells and possibly predispose them to become cancerous).

antitumor effect. Activity against cancer cells.

anxiety. An uncomfortable feeling of worry, uneasiness, or dread; a normal reaction to the perception of a threat to one's body, lifestyle, values, or loved ones.

ascites. Abnormal accumulation of fluid in the abdomen.

asymptomatic. Without symptoms.

atrophy. Wasting or decrease in the size of a part of the body.

atypical. Unusual, not ordinary, not normal, such as an atypical course for Hodgkin's disease or an atypical reaction to Adriamycin (a type of chemotherapy).

autologous transplant. Removal of a patient's tissue, such as bone marrow, and its return to the same patient after cancer treatment. For example, a patient may have bone marrow removed, then the bone marrow is treated in the test tube while the patient receives cancer treatment in the hospital, after which the treated bone marrow is returned to the same patient.

axilla. Armpit.

B cell. One type of cell in the humoral, antibody-forming immune system; a type of lymphocyte.

benign tumor. An abnormal growth that is not a cancer. It cannot spread to other parts of the body but can create problems because of its location.

beta-carotene. A pigment that is a precursor to vitamin A; one of a group of substances that acts as an antioxidant in the body.

bilateral. On both sides of the body.

biofeedback. A technique based on the principle that you can change your body or your behavior more effectively if you have information (feedback) on how close you are to your goal.

biological response modifiers. Agents that stimulate the patient's immune system to kill cancer cells, e.g., interferon, interleukin-2, and LAK cells.

blastic. An X ray finding of a bone that shows more calcium than normal.

blood–brain barrier. The system of cells that prevents infection and medicines from getting into the central nervous system.

bone marrow. Soft substance in the center of bones; the place where blood cells are made.

BSE. Breast self-exam.

Cancer. A general term for over 200 diseases characterized by an abnormal and uncontrolled malignant growth of cells. The mass, or tumor, can invade and destroy surrounding normal tissues. The cancer cells can spread through the blood or lymph system to start new cancers in other parts of the body.

candida. A type of yeast (fungus), also called monilia.

carcinogen. Something that causes or increases the risk of developing cancer in animals or humans.

carcinoma. A cancer that begins in tissue that lines an organ or duct.

carcinoma in situ. A very early stage of cancer, where it is confined to a small area.

cardiac. Related to the heart.

carotenoid. A substance (a pigment) that contains carotene, a precursor to vitamin A.

cell. The unit structure of all living tissue.

cellulitis. Inflammation of the skin.

central nervous system. The brain and spinal cord.

cervical. Related to the neck of any structure; most often referring to either the tip of the female uterus which protrudes into the vagina (such as cervical cancer), or the region of the neck between the head and the shoulders (such as a cervical disk or a cervical lymph node). Note that this term refers to one of two completely different parts of the body.

cervix. The portion of the uterus that projects into the vagina.

chemoprevention (chemoprophylaxis). Treatment aimed at preventing the development of cancer.

chemosurgery. The use of drugs applied to the skin to kill skin cancer cells.

chemotherapy. Treatment with anticancer drugs.

clinical. Pertaining to work with people (as opposed to lab studies with test tubes or animals).

clinical trials. Investigational studies in people of new cancer treatments.

cognition. Awareness with reasoning, judgment, and memory; normally functioning thinking.

colostomy. An artificial opening in the abdominal wall to drain colon contents into a bag.

contraindicated. Related to a situation in which a treatment cannot be used because specific symptoms or circumstances make the risks too great.

conventional therapy. Standard treatment whose effectiveness has been well established by sound scientific studies.

cruciferous vegetables. Cauliflower, brussels sprouts, cabbage, and other vegetables that are rich in beta-carotene.

cryosurgery. Surgery by means of an instrument that freezes the tissue.

cure (for cancer). A condition in which there is no evidence of cancer and the person has the same life expectancy as if he or she had never had cancer. Each different type of cancer requires a specific length of time without evidence of cancer before the person is considered cured. For many cancers the time is five years; for some it is only one to two years. Some cancers are considered incurable because, no matter how many years without evidence of recurrent cancer, the person always has a greater chance of developing that type of cancer again than if he or she had never had cancer (recurrences for that type of cancer occur with some regularity after five, ten, twenty, or more years). Cure is not a guarantee against recurrence; cure means that your chance of recurrence is the same as your chance for developing that type of cancer if you had never had cancer before.

cyst. A sac containing fluid and/or solid material; it is usually benign, but can be malignant.

cytotoxin. An agent that kills cells.

debulking. A procedure to remove as much cancer as possible; reducing the "bulk" of the cancer.

delayed complications. Medical problems that may occur weeks or months (sometimes years) after the completion of treatment and that are due to the cancer or the treatment itself.

delayed effects. Expected changes that are measurable weeks to months (sometimes years) after the cancer treatment and that are due to the cancer or the treatment itself.

diuretic. A medicine given in order to eliminate salt and water from the body.

dose-limiting. Drawing a limit on how much of a certain treatment can be given. For example, each area of the body can receive only a certain total amount of radiation, and each individual can receive only a certain total amount of specific chemotherapeutic agents in his or her lifetime without serious side effects.

drug resistance. The development of resistance to cancer drugs by cancer cells, or to antibiotics by bacteria.

durable power of attorney. A legal document specifying someone (a "proxy") who will make health care decisions in the event that the person in question becomes unable to make decisions.

durable remission. Remission that lasts a long time; not the same as cure.

edema. Fluid accumulation; swelling due to fluid.

esophageal speech. A form of intelligible sound used by people who have had their voice box removed; speech created by moving air a special way up the esophagus.

esophagitis. Irritation or inflammation of the esophagus caused by infection, radiation, chemotherapy, acid reflux, or other injury.

esophagus. The digestive tube connecting the mouth and the stomach.

faint. Loss of consciousness as a result of insufficient blood to the brain.

fine-needle aspiration. Use of a needle to obtain a biopsy (a piece of tissue) through the skin.

fissures. Cracks in the skin or a membrane.

fistula. An abnormal opening or connection between one part of the body and another, or between the inside of the body and the outside.

frozen section. A preliminary reading of a biopsy specimen, available within minutes to hours of obtaining the tissue. Final, definitive results are usually available after the "permanent sections" are read, which may be days to weeks later.

gene. A unit of DNA; the basic unit of heredity.

gene probe. A laboratory tool that identifies an abnormality in the genes of a tumor cell or a normal cell; this abnormality is thought to be related to the development of a cancer cell.

grade (of a cancer). A descriptive term referring to how aggressive the cancer cells appear under the microscope.

graft versus host disease. A medical complication of bone marrow transplantation or of blood transfusion received from a different person, whereby the patient's immune system tries to reject the foreign marrow or blood.

guaiac test. Also called hemoccult; a sensitive test for detecting microscopic blood in the stool, used to screen for colon cancer. A number of factors can cause the result to indicate blood when there is, in fact, none (a "false positive") or indicate the absence of blood when there is, in fact, blood (a "false negative"). The test can indicate blood resulting from any blood source from the mouth to the anus (such as a stomach ulcer or a noncancerous vessel that is leaking).

gynecomastia. Breast enlargement in men, usually seen as a side effect of certain medications or as a complication of certain cancers.

heart block. A condition when the heart does not beat regularly, because of an abnormality of its electrical conduction system.

heart failure. The condition when the heart does not pump blood adequately; can cause fluid buildup in the lungs, as well as other problems.

heart murmur. An abnormal sound heard through a stethoscope and produced by blood flowing through the heart.

hepatic. Related to the liver.

hepatotoxic. Damaging to the liver.

herpes zoster (shingles). A painful skin rash caused by reactivation of chicken pox virus.

histology. The appearance of tissue under the microscope.

Hodgkin's disease. A type of cancer of the lymph system; a type of lymphoma.

hormone. A substance released by (endocrine) glands that affects parts of the body away from the gland.

hospice care. Care whose focus is physical, emotional, and spiritual comfort, usually without further anticancer treatment; care instituted when life expectancy is short (e.g., less than six months).

hyperplasia. Increased number of cells; not necessarily cancer.

hyperthyroid. Marked by too high a level of thyroid hormone.

hypothyroid. Marked by too low a level of thyroid hormone.

immune system. White blood cells and antibodies that protect the body by attacking foreign substances.

immunology. The branch of science dealing with the body's system for resistance to disease and rejection of foreign substances.

immunosuppression. Lowered immunity causing lowered ability to fight infection and disease.

immunosuppressives (immunosuppressive medicine). Drugs that cause the immune system to be less active.

immunotherapy. Cancer therapy that stimulates the body's own immune system to kill cancer cells.

impotence. Inability in the male to have sexual intercourse, i.e., to achieve or sustain an erection.

incontinence. Loss of ability to control urination (urinary incontinence) or defecation (fecal incontinence).

infarction. Death of an area of tissue (such as in the heart or the brain) as a result of an interruption of blood supply to the area.

infection. The condition when a part of the body or the entire body is invaded by an agent that causes disease, such as a virus, bacteria, or fungus.

inflammation. A body tissue reaction to injury that usually causes pain, swelling, redness, and decreased function.

informed consent. Competent and voluntary permission to go ahead with a procedure or treatment.

interferons. Proteins produced by the body in small amounts to help fight viral infection; interferons are also produced artificially and injected in larger amounts as one type of cancer treatment.

invasive cancer. Cancer that has spread from its original site to the surrounding healthy tissue.

jaundice. Yellowing of the skin, whites of the eyes, mucus membranes, and body fluids because of an accumulation of bile pigment; a sign of liver disease, but can be caused by certain blood disorders, too.

job lock. The situation when a person cannot leave a job without risking losing his or her insurance coverage, and the person has or had a medical condition that will make it difficult to obtain new insurance, or when a person cannot leave a job without losing insurance for a family member who will have difficulty getting new coverage.

laparotomy. Surgery that opens the abdomen.

larynx. The part of the windpipe that contains the voice box.

laser. A concentrated beam of light that destroys with heat anything in its path.

late complications. Medical problems as a result of cancer or treatment that occur sometimes, are not expected, and appear months to years following cancer treatment.

late effects. Changes or medical problems that occur months to years after completion of cancer treatment and are due to the cancer or treatment.

leukemia. Cancer of the white blood cells.

leukopenia. Low white blood cell count.

libido. Sexual drive, conscious or unconscious.

light-headedness. The feeling of being about to faint or "black out"; caused by inadequate circulation to the brain.

living will. A written document that outlines what a patient would want or not want done to prolong his or her life artificially (with medicines and machines) if critically ill with little chance of recovery.

localized. Limited to the site of origin, no evidence of spread.

lymph. Clear fluid formed throughout the body, which flows in the lymphatic system, is filtered in the lymph nodes, and then is added to the blood. It carries infection-fighting cells.

lymphatic system. A circulation system, like the blood system, that carries lymph throughout the body. The lymph organs include the lymph nodes, spleen, and thymus.

lymphoma. Cancer of the lymphatic system.

lymph nodes. Rounded bean-shaped organs that make some of the white blood cells (lymphocytes and monocytes) and filter the lymph before it enters the blood. Their size varies from that of a pinhead to that of an olive. There are thousands of them throughout the body, the most obvious ones being in the neck (cervical lymph nodes), the armpit (axillary lymph nodes), and the groin (inguinal lymph nodes). They may become cancerous themselves (lymphoma) or be a place to which cancer spreads (such as metastic lung cancer).

lymphedema. Swelling caused by obstruction of the lymph vessels.

lymphocytes. White blood cells that make antibodies and destroy infections and cancer cells.

lytic. An X-ray finding in a bone that shows less calcium than normal.

markers (tumor markers). Chemicals in the blood that indicate the possibility of cancer, used in the diagnosis or follow-up of cancer.

melanoma. A form of skin cancer that often arises from a mole.

metastasis (metastases, plural). The spread of cancer cells from their original site.

metastasize. To spread.

monoclonal antibodies. A new technique being investigated for diagnosing and treating certain types of cancer that involves very specific antibodies that will react with the cancer cells.

morbidity. The state of being sick or diseased.

mortality. Death rate.

mucositis. Inflammation of the linings of the mouth.

multimodality. A technique using two or more types of therapy, such as surgery and radiation.

myeloma (multiple myeloma). Cancer of the plasma cells that starts in the bone marrow.

narcotic. Any addictive drug (such as morphine or codeine) that blunts or distorts the senses and induces sleep; a drug that in moderate doses lessens or relieves pain and produces sleepiness or sleep, but that in excessive doses causes unconsciousness, coma, and possibly death.

necrosis. Dead tissue; can be caused by chemotherapy, radiation, heat, infection, or lack of circulation.

neoadjuvant chemotherapy. Therapy given before surgery or radiation therapy in the hope of decreasing the tumor burden and also killing cancer cells that may be missed by subsequent surgery or radiation.

neoplasm. A tumor, abnormal growth of tissue; may be benign or malignant.

nephrotoxic. Damaging to the kidneys.

neuropathy. Malfunction or disease of a nerve (or nerves).

neurosis. Anxiety that leads to maladaptive coping tools that result in abnormal behavior or symptoms.

neurotoxic. Damaging to the nervous system.

no code. A directive written in the hospital or home nursing chart not to try to resuscitate a patient whose heart stops or who stops breathing; also called "DNR" (do not resuscitate).

nodule. Lump, tumor; may be benign or malignant.

obstruction. Blockage.

oncogenes. Genes involved in the development of cancer cells.

oncologist. A doctor specializing in cancer diagnosis and treatment.

oncology. The branch of medicine dealing with cancer.

oophorectomy. Surgical removal of one or both ovaries.

opportunistic infections. Unusual infections that occur in people with weakened immune systems. Healthy people who are exposed to the same infectious agents rarely get sick, because the well-functioning immune system prevents illness.

ostomy. Surgical opening in the skin, allowing connection to an internal organ for drainage.

ototoxicity. Damage to the hearing system.

palliative. Treatment for comfort, not cure. Anticancer drugs or radiation can be used to control the cancer, and thereby control pain, but the treatment is not intended to cure the patient.

palpation. Examination with the hands to determine shape, size, texture, consistency, location.

paresthesia. Skin sensation of burning, tingling, prickling.

Patient Self-Determination Act. A federal law that requires that patients be informed about their rights under state law to accept or refuse treatment, as well as help patients execute a living will and appoint a medical proxy if they so wish.

pathological fracture. A broken bone that occurs after minimal trauma or with normal activity because the bone is weakened by disease such as cancer.

pathologist. A doctor who specializes in diagnosing disease by looking at tissue directly, under the microscope, and with other technology.

pathology. The study of disease; condition produced by disease.

perioperative. Around the time of surgery.

peritoneum. The lining of the abdominal cavity.

pharmacology. The study of drugs.

pharynx. The upper throat.

phlebitis. Inflammation of a vein.

photosensitivity. Increased skin sensitivity to the sun.

placebo. A treatment designed to have no therapeutic effect, such as a sugar pill or a saltwater intravenous drip.

platelet. A type of blood cell that is involved in clotting (preventing and stopping bleeding).

polyp. A growth from a mucous membrane that can become cancerous.

primary cancer. Place where the cancer first started.

proctoscopy. Evaluation of the rectum with a scope.

progesterone. A female hormone.

prognosis. Prediction of how well the patient will do.

prophylactic. Preventive.

prosthesis. An artificial replacement for a missing body part.

protocol. Description of the treatment steps (the "recipe").

proxy. A person appointed to make medical decisions for another person in the event that the latter becomes unable to make health care decisions.

pulmonary. Related to the lungs.

radiation therapy. Treatment by means of radioactive substances.

radiologist. A doctor specializing in the taking and interpretation of X rays, CAT scans, and MRI scans. Some radiologists are trained in the treatment of disease with X ray–guided therapy ("interventional radiologists").

radioresistent. Cells resistant to the effects of radiation.

radiosensitive. Sensitive to radiation; said especially of cancer cells that are killed by it.

radiotherapist (radiation oncologist). A physician who specializes in the treatment of disease by means of radiation therapy.

recurrence. Reappearance of the same cancer after a period when there was no evidence of cancer.

regional involvement. Cancer that is limited to one area of the body; regional treatment is limited to one area of the body.

regression (of cancer). Shrinkage of tumor.

rehabilitation. Treatment and education aimed at healing and adjusting to the changes brought on by disease and treatment; treatment aimed at enabling the disabled patient to be as independent and self-fulfilled as possible.

relapse. Return of symptoms after improvement; return of cancer (recurrence).

remission. Partial or complete shrinkage of cancer.

renal. Related to the kidney.

resect. Cut off or remove.

resectable. Able to be removed.

residual disease (or cancer, or tumor). Remaining cancer after treatment.

resistance. Failure of the disease or problem to respond to treatment.

respiratory. Related to the breathing system.

restaging. Evaluation after treatment is completed, to see how much cancer is left.

retroperitoneum. The space behind the abdominal cavity.

risk factors (for cancer). Conditions or habits that increase one's chance of developing cancer.

salvage. Attempt to cure after earlier attempts have failed.

sarcoma. Cancer of the soft tissue (muscles, nerves, tendons, blood vessels) or bones.

screening. Evaluation for early disease when there are no symptoms.

second-look surgery. Surgery done as part of reevaluation after completion of treatment to determine whether any cancer is left.

sepsis. Infection in the blood.

shingles. See *herpes zoster.*

side effect. The secondary effect of a treatment; reaction to treatment other than the curative effects.

sigmoidoscopy. Examination of the lower colon by means of a scope equipped with fiberoptics.

soporific. A substance inducing sleep.

spleen. An organ in the left upper abdomen that is part of the lymphatic system; it helps to remove old red blood cells, produce white blood cells, and store blood.

sputum. Phlegm; mucus from the lungs and bronchial airways.

stable. Unchanged; not worse nor better.

staging. Evaluation to see how far the cancer has spread.

stereotactic needle biopsy. Biopsy with a needle where the needle is guided by X ray or CAT scan pictures.

stilbestrol. A synthetic female hormone.

stomatitis. Irritation of the mouth.

supplemental therapy. Treatment intended to be used in addition to conventional therapy, such as visual imagery, special diets, vitamins, exercise, counseling, prayer, humor, and biofeedback.

suppository. Medication administered into the rectum.

survivor (cancer survivor). Anyone diagnosed with cancer who is alive, from the time of the discovery of cancer and for the balance of life.

susceptibility testing. A branch of genetic counseling that determines a person's susceptibility to cancer (risk of getting cancer) on the basis of an analysis of disease in family members.

systemic. Involving the entire body.

T cell. A type of cell involved in the cellular immune system; a type of lymphocyte.

teratogen. An agent that causes birth defects if the mother is exposed to it while pregnant.

terminal. Referring to a condition for which curative treatment is unavailable, life expectancy is short, and further treatment to control the cancer is not available. (The intention of this term should be clarified in discussions that use it.)

tissue. A group of similar cells, such as lung tissue, brain tissue, lymph node tissue.

titrate. Adjust the dose of treatment; fine-tune the dose of treatment.

TNM classification. A system for assigning the stage of most kinds of cancer (not used for lymphomas and leukemias).

tolerance. A person's ability to handle the effects of a treatment; increasing ability to handle the same or increased amount of treatment.

toxic. Resembling or caused by a poison.

TPN (total parenteral nutrition). Complete nourishment through intravenous access (in the veins).

tumor. Abnormal mass of tissue that may be either benign or malignant (cancerous).

tumor necrosis factor (TNF). Protein produced by certain white blood cells in response to certain bacteria that has been found to help kill cancer cells.

tumor registry. A hospital-based person or group who collects information about people who have been diagnosed or treated for cancer at the hospital; the bank of information on cancer patients who are treated at a particular hospital or clinic.

ulcer. A breakdown in the surface lining (skin ulcer, stomach ulcer, duodenal ulcer).

unilateral. On one side of the body.

venipuncture. Puncture of the vein for any purpose, such as getting a blood sample or administering medicine.

vertigo. Sensation of moving or other things moving around despite being still; dizziness.

vital signs. A group of measurements including temperature, blood pressure, pulse, and rate of breathing; may include body weight and height.

vitamins. Compounds that are essential in small quantities for health.

workup. Total evaluation of a patient including a physical exam, blood tests, scans, and discussions.

APPENDIX II

—

Annotated Bibliography

UNDERSTANDING THE MEDICINE OF RECOVERY FROM CANCER TREATMENT AND SPECIFIC AFTEREFFECTS OF CANCER TREATMENT (CHAPTERS 1 AND 2)

Oncology is a rapidly changing field. People who are interested in learning more about cancer must make sure their information is up-to-date and accurate. Statistics and specific facts about recovery and aftereffects of cancer treatment may be misleading if the book is already a few years old, because it considers treatments that may have given way to safer, more reliable ones.

A number of books that deal with the medicine of cancer include brief mention of or sections on the medicine of recovery and aftereffects of cancer treatment. Susan Nessim and Judith Ellis, *Cancervive: The Challenge of Life after Cancer* (Boston: Houghton Mifflin, 1991), is devoted to a discussion of the medicine and emotions of remission. Written by a layperson survivor, the medical sections are brief and general. Nessim includes an informative table of medical follow-up guidelines for long-term effects. Malin Dollinger, M.D., et al., *Everyone's Guide to Cancer Therapy: How Cancer Is Diagnosed, Treated, and Managed Day to Day* (Kansas City, Mo., and New York: Andrews and McMeel, 1991), is an excellent comprehensive resource written for the layperson. The last section of the book reviews each of the common cancers and outlines a strategy for treatment follow-up, the treatment for recurrence, and a list of the most important questions you can ask. Marion Morra and Eva Potts, *Choices: Realistic Alternatives in Cancer Treatment* (New York: Avon Books, 1987), is another comprehensive resource for the layperson, written in question-and-answer format. Information about issues related to recovery is integrated throughout the text. However, there is no easy way to separate out this information, because it is not assigned to any particular section of each chapter.

Two well-respected works are Vincent T. DeVita, Jr., et al., *Cancer: Principles and Practice of Oncology,* 3rd ed. (Philadelphia: J. B. Lippincott, 1990), and A. R. Moossa et al., *Comprehensive Textbook of Oncology,* 2nd ed. (Baltimore: Williams and Wilkins, 1991). These mammoth volumes are medical textbooks aimed at the physician. They are written in technical language and assume a sophisticated medical background. Their strength lies in their comprehensiveness and well-accepted information. Their main drawback is that by the time a text goes to press, it is outdated in regard to investigational approaches and available data analyzing comparative efficiency and safety of treatment options. Books can be supplemented with oncology journals, available for review in medical school and some hospital libraries. Librarians can help you locate articles appropriate to your specific questions. These articles tend to be quite technical and sophisticated.

Cancer Facts and Figures is an annual report available from the American Cancer Society (ACS), which also puts out *Unproven Methods of Treatment.*

PRACTICAL ISSUES (Chapter 3)

Nessim's *Cancervive* deals with practical issues of recovery in a sensitive and helpful manner. She discusses insurance issues, job lock and other work-related problems, infertility, and so forth. *Charting the Journey: An Almanac of Practical Resources for Cancer Survivors,* edited by Fitzhugh Mullan, M.D., Barbara Hoffman, J.D., and the editors of Consumer Reports Books (New York: Consumers Union, 1990), was devised by the National Coalition for Cancer Survivorship. It is written in clear language for the layperson, focusing on the practical aspects of surviving; it includes a discussion of legal, financial, and insurance problems that affect the survivor after completion of cancer treatment. The table of contents and index make the information easily accessible. Danette G. Kauffman, *Surviving Cancer: A Practical Guide for Those Fighting to Win* (Washington, D.C.: Acropolis, 1989), deals with practical and emotional issues of cancer. A unique strength of this book is the thorough listing of resources at the end of each section, which is useful not only for the newly diagnosed patient but for the patient who has completed therapy as well.

EMOTIONAL ISSUES OF SURVIVORSHIP (Chapter 4)

William V. Pietsch, *The Serenity Prayer Book* (New York: HarperSanFrancisco, 1990), is a beautifully written interpretation of the popular prayer of recovering alcoholics. It offers a profoundly comforting foundation for dealing with recovery from cancer treatment, as well as a healthy way to live with or without cancer. *Cancervive* discusses many of the universal issues of survivorship in a sensitive and hopeful way. David Spiegel's *Living beyond Limits* (New York: Times Books, 1993) is must reading for anyone interested in scientifically sound information and advice about the role of the mind–body connection in illness and healing. In his clear, concise, and readable style, Dr. Spiegel nourishes hope and facilitates healing by exposing popular theories about the mind–body connection that hurt rather than help and by encouraging people to believe that they can learn how to live beyond the limits of their illness. *Spinning Straw into Gold* (New York: Simon and Schuster, 1991) is written by Ronnie Kaye, a psychotherapist who survived breast cancer. Even though it is about recovery from breast cancer, most of the emotional issues apply to survivors of any type of cancer. Of all the dozens of books written about coping with the emotional aftermath of a cancer diagnosis, Kaye's is particularly clear and insightful, offering tools that may help you and your family adjust. Arthur Frank's *At the Will of the Body* (Boston: Houghton Mifflin, 1991) is a profound reflection on the dynamics of illness. Pesach Krauss, *Why Me? Coping with Grief, Loss, and Change* (New York: Bantam Books, 1988), is a powerful book with a religious slant. Susan Sontag's seminal work *Illness as Metaphor* (New York: Vintage Books, 1979) exposes the myths surrounding cancer. Daniel Rosenblum, M.D., *A Time to Hear, a Time to Help* (New York: Free Press, 1993), sensitively presents issues involving cancer doctors and their patients and through anecdotes explores the dynamics of this special relationship. Ernest Lawrence Rossi's *The Psychobiology of Mind–*

Body Healing: New Concepts of Therapeutic Hypnosis (New York: W. W. Norton, 1986) is a thorough yet concise review of the scientific evidence for the mind–body connection. It is a bit dry but worth a close reading, especially its approach to using that connection for self-healing. Two books that deal with the healing effect of humor and pleasure are Allen Klein's *The Healing Power of Humor* (Los Angeles: Jeremy P. Tarcher, 1989) and Robert Ornstein and David Sobel's *Healthy Pleasures* (Reading, Mass.: Addison-Wesley, 1989).

APPENDIX III

———

Resources for the Patient Who Has Completed Cancer Treatment

NCI (NATIONAL CANCER INSTITUTE)

The National Cancer Institute provides a Cancer Information Service (CIS). 1-800-4CANCER is a toll-free number answered by trained volunteers, who are prepared to deal with questions about cancer or to direct you to the place or person who can give you answers. The NCI has a large number of informational booklets, which you can obtain free of charge, by calling the toll-free number above.

After you complete your treatments, you may want to request information on current recommendations regarding prevention of recurrence and of second cancers. If you are interested in staying up-to-date regarding ongoing clinical trials for your type of cancer, the NCI can provide listings of those trials registered with them. Clinical trials constitute one type of information available through NCI's "PDQ" (Physician Data Query), a frequently updated review of recommended treatment for most types of cancer, available clinical trials, and lists of doctors and hospitals.

The NCI also provides, on request, a listing of the nation's comprehensive cancer centers. These centers research and study new methods of diagnosis, treatment, and prevention of cancer, as well as provide teaching and patient care. In addition, the NCI can supply a list of the nation's clinical cancer centers, which conduct NCI-supported research on cancer diagnosis and treatment.

Some of the information provided by this service is available by fax machine. "CancerFax" allows you to request information about your type of cancer, the current recommendations for treatment, and a list of free patient publications available from the Office of Cancer Communications. Available twenty-four hours a day, seven days a week, it can be reached by dialing 1-301-402-5874 from a fax machine. Voice prompts will direct you to the desired information.

AMERICAN CANCER SOCIETY (ACS)

The American Cancer Society is a nationwide community-based voluntary organization with national and local offices. You can obtain the telephone number of the local office from your oncologist or the yellow pages. The ACS has trained volunteers, many of whom have dealt with cancer themselves, to answer questions, provide informational pamphlets and videos, and offer personal or group support.

The ACS can serve as a source of information about recovery from treatment, prevention of second cancers, information and support in coping with such changes as loss of your voice (International Association of Laryngectomees), loss of your breast (Reach to Recovery), or an ostomy (Ostomy Rehabilitation Program) or with the overall experience of surviving your type of cancer (CanSurmount). Many local units of the ACS offer support or self-help groups. Their national office is

> American Cancer Society (ACS)
> National Headquarters
> 1599 Clifton Rd, N.E.
> Atlanta, GA 30329
> 404-320-3333

The Canadian Cancer Society (CCS) offers many of the same services as the American Cancer Society. The location and telephone number of provincial divisions is listed in the telephone directory. Their national office is

Canadian Cancer Society
130 Bloor Street West
Suite 1001
Toronto, Ontario
Canada M5S 2V7
416-961-7223

As you get far enough away from your own experience with cancer, you may wish to share your knowledge, experience, and energy with recently diagnosed patients and their families. The ACS provides one vehicle for helping others.

NATIONAL COALITION FOR CANCER SURVIVORSHIP (NCCS)

The National Coalition for Cancer Survivorship is a growing movement, focusing on issues of importance to cancer survivors after completion of treatments. It publishes a quarterly newsletter, *The Networker,* offering the latest news about concerns that affect survivors. *Facing Forward,* published in collaboration with the National Cancer Institute, is a guide for those who have finished treatment. A bibliography on insurance and employment concerns of cancer survivors, a bibliography of "Best Loved Books," and many kinds of cancer survivorship information are available. The NCCS also provides guidance or assistance to resolve insurance and employment problems and to locate local cancer support groups and services. You can obtain everything by writing or calling

National Coalition for Cancer Survivorship (NCCS)
1010 Wayne Avenue, Fifth Floor
Silver Spring, MD 20910
301-650-8868

SOCIAL SERVICES

The social service department of your local hospital is usually well informed about all the services available in your community (support groups, local supply stores, local support services, local treatment facilities). Experts in the issues of survivorship after completion of treatment may be available for individual or group consultation or counseling. They may be a good resource to help you deal with ongoing medical, emotional, or social difficulties.

THE OFFICE OF YOUR ONCOLOGIST

The staff of your oncologist is familiar with most of the needs and problems that you will face after completion of treatment. Even though you may be through with cancer treatment, your questions, concerns, and needs are important.

LATE EFFECTS CLINICS

A growing number of hospitals and medical centers have established late effects clinics, which focus on the issues and problems of long-term survivorship. Specialists at these clinics may provide further information about late effects or a second opinion on the evaluation and treatment of a specific problem.

> Post-Treatment Resource Program
> Memorial Sloan-Kettering Cancer Center
> 410 East 62nd Street
> New York, NY 10021
> 212-639-3292

Call your local hospitals and your local office of the American Cancer Society to find out whether they have any programs geared to the cancer survivor who has completed treatments.

APPENDIX IV

Understanding the Different Types of Health Care Workers

A number of different doctors have participated in the evaluation and treatment of your cancer. Most likely, a surgeon or specialist performed your biopsy or a subsequent surgery, a pathologist read and interpreted the biopsy, and an oncologist (cancer specialist) prescribed and supervised your treatment. You may have been cared for by doctors in training and general practitioners, as well as by highly specialized physicians.

After the completion of cancer treatment, medical problems may persist or develop. Evaluating or treating these problems may involve additional specialists or nonphysician health care professionals. Understanding their role will make your evaluation and treatment less confusing and enable you to participate in key decisions. If your internist or oncologist does not recommend consultation with a specialist and you want a second opinion about a problem or decision, you may request a referral. He or she may proceed with the referral or explain why this is unnecessary or inappropriate in your case. Many specialists require a referral from a physician before they will see you. As in all other aspects of your care, you have a right to a second opinion.

Here is a listing of most of the health care professionals and their areas of expertise. There is considerable overlap, with different specialists having expertise in similar areas. When two or more treat the same problem, the referral to one of them will depend on the presumed cause of your problem or the expected treatment that will be needed. You may have to see a series of specialists before the cause or your problem is clarified or optimum treatment is obtained.

Doctors often indicate that they are "board-certified." This indicates that they have completed a required training program (three to five years, depending on the specialty) and have passed rigorous examinations designed by other doctors who practice the particular specialty. It offers you some assurance of medical competence, although it says little about the doctor's bedside manner or diligence in keeping up-to-date. There are many well-qualified doctors who are not board-certified, because they went into practice before the specialty boards were established.

You are urged to continue your care with your primary care physician (see listing below) or to establish yourself with one. The chief advantage of having a primary general doctor, such as an internist or family practitioner, is that you have someone who knows all about you. When your primary care physician evaluates any problem, big or little, all of your past and current medical problems are taken into account, as well as your family history, personality, social situation, and coping style.

PRIMARY CARE MEDICAL DOCTORS

These are doctors who have received training in all broad areas of medicine. They evaluate and treat all organ systems as well as pay attention to psychosocial issues. They oversee your routine care, supervise the evaluation and treatment of any medical problems, determine when the expertise of a specialist is needed, and serve as a resource of information and support when specific problems are addressed by specialists.

Everyone should have a primary care doctor because he or she will know about your past and present problems and can coordinate all of your health care needs. Primary care doctors can help ensure that you follow routine health maintenance and preventive measures and can be your first contact when you develop problems or have questions.

Like a marriage, a working relationship with your primary care physician is long-term and develops over time. You come to know which problems your primary care doctor will evaluate and treat and which ones require the expertise of a specialist, when to call your primary care doctor and when to call one of your other doctors. When in doubt, contact your primary care physician first. It is your responsibility to keep your primary care doctor apprised of your medical condition, especially if a specialist evaluates a new problem or makes changes in your medications.

A *family practitioner* is a doctor who is board-certified in the comprehensive medical care of people of all ages and in the diagnosis and treatment of diseases and disorders of all organ systems. Family practitioners are trained in the medicine of pregnancy, delivery, and after delivery (obstetrics), gynecology, internal medicine, pediatrics, psychiatry, and surgery. Family practitioners diagnose and treat problems, counsel, and coordinate the patient's total health care.

A *general practitioner* is a doctor whose training is similar to, if not the same as, that of a family practitioner but who is not board-certified in family practice. Often this is because he or she completed training before the establishment of family practice as a separate entity.

A *geriatrician* is a doctor who specializes in the evaluation and treatment of medical problems of elderly people (generally older than sixty-five years).

A *gynecologist* is a doctor who specializes in diseases and disorders of the female reproductive organs, including the breasts. Although specialists, they often serve as primary care physicians to women who do not have any other doctors. However, they have not received the same training as the other primary care practitioners in the evaluation and treatment of diseases and disorders outside of the reproductive organ system.

An *internist* is a doctor who specializes in diseases and disorders of the internal organs of adults by other than surgical means. Internists are trained in the evaluation and treatment of diseases of every organ system, the evaluation and approach to psychosocial issues, counseling, and coordinating patients' total health care.

A *pediatrician* is a doctor who specializes in the evaluation and treatment of medical problems of babies, youngsters, adolescents, and young adults.

MEDICAL SPECIALISTS

Specialists are doctors who have received additional training in certain areas and who treat diseases with medicines. They may be skilled in performing invasive procedures, such as a spinal tap or a biopsy through a fiber-optic tube (colonscope, bronchoscope, etc.), but do not perform major surgery. Most of these specialties feature individual doctors who are additionally specialized in that they treat only children (pediatric gastroenterologist, pediatric neurologist, and so on).

An *allergist* is a doctor who evaluates and treats diseases and disorders of the immune system that cause reactions to substances that do not normally cause a reaction, diseases such as asthma, eczema, rhinitis (runny nose), hay fever, urticaria (hives), and food allergy. Symptoms that may prompt referral to an allergist include wheezing, shortness of breath, persistent cough, rashes, irritation of eyes, swelling of the eyes, nose, mouth, or throat, fainting after exposure to foods or other substances, and known allergy to certain drugs and the need to be desensitized in order to take them.

An *anesthesiologist* is a doctor trained in techniques that cause the patient to have partial or complete loss of sensation with or without the loss of consciousness. Anesthesia is accomplished with the use of medications, surgical techniques, or mechanical techniques. Some anesthesiologists are trained to treat pain syndromes. Symptoms that may prompt referral to an anesthesiologist who specializes in the treatment of pain syndromes include burning, aching, and sharp or dull pain.

A *cardiologist* is a doctor who evaluates and treats diseases and disorders of the cardiovascular (heart and circulation) system, such as coronary artery disease (hardening of the arteries that feed the heart), cardiomyopathy (disease of the heart muscle itself, such as occurs with alcoholism, after radiation to the heart, or with chronic disease of the small vessels to the heart), hypertension (high blood pressure), heart valve disease, hyperlipidemia (e.g., high cholesterol), infection of the heart, heart failure, heart rhythm abnormalities, heart murmurs, phlebitis (inflammation of a vein), and peripheral arterial disease (hardening or blockage of an artery to the arm, leg, bowel, or other region). Symptoms that may prompt referral include palpitations, fainting, loss of consciousness, leg swelling, cold painful feet, shortness of breath when lying flat, wheezing, unexplained fever, stroke, or exercise-induced chest pain or heaviness, shortness of breath, and aching in the jaw or arm or leg.

A *dermatologist* is a doctor who evaluates and treats diseases of the skin, such as skin cancer, urticaria (hives), acne, psoriasis, eczema, seborrhea, cellulitis (skin infection), fungal infections, herpes simplex, herpes zoster (shingles), warts, and burns. Symptoms that may prompt referral include rashes, itching, and changes in pigmentation.

An *endocrinologist* is a doctor who evaluates and treats diseases and disorders of the glands that produce hormones, including diabetes, high or low thyroid, high or low calcium, and high or low adrenalin. Symptoms that may prompt referral include weight change, heat or cold intolerance, excessive urination, a lump in your thyroid gland, excessive fatigue, and a change in menses (menstrual periods).

An *ENT ("ear-nose-throat doctor," otolaryngologist)* is a doctor who evaluates and treats diseases and disorders of the ear, nose, and throat. Symptoms that may prompt referral include a change in hearing, ringing in the ears, vertigo, sinus headaches, postnasal drip, sore throats, a lump in the head or neck areas, nosebleeds, facial pain, and a change in voice.

A *gynecologist* is a doctor of the female reproductive system, including the breasts, with expertise in evaluating and treating problems related to "female hormones." Symptoms that may prompt referral to a gynecologist include subfertility or infertility, vaginal pain or discharge, irregular menses (periods), breast tenderness or pain, and altered sex drive.

A *gastroenterologist* is a doctor who evaluates and treats diseases and disorders of the digestive tract (stomach, intestines, esophagus, liver, gallbladder, pancreas), such as colitis, esophagitis, stomach or duodenal ulcers, hepatitis, malnutrition, jaundice, hemorrhoids, gallstones, liver failure, and cirrhosis. Symptoms that may prompt referral include nausea, vomiting, weight loss, rectal bleeding, abdominal pain, difficulty swallowing, chest pain, anemia, jaundice (yellow skin and eyes), diarrhea, constipation, and heartburn.

A *hematologist* is a doctor who evaluates and treats diseases and disorders of the blood, such as anemia, polycythemia, and clotting factor deficiencies. Symptoms that may prompt referral include anemia (low red blood cell count) and abnormal bleeding (bleeding or clotting too easily). Most hematologists combine specializations in hematology and oncology (cancer medicine) and are called hematologist-oncologists.

An *infectious disease specialist* is a doctor who diagnoses, treats, and prevents illness caused by infectious agents such as bacteria, fungi, and viruses. Infectious diseases include tuberculosis, venereal disease, candida (yeast), Lyme's disease, pneumonia, meningitis, cellulitis (skin infection), osteomyelitis (bone infection), and hepatitis (liver infection).

Symptoms that may prompt referral include persistent fatigue, fevers, nonhealing skin lesions or bone pain, weight loss, diarrhea, and coughing.

An infertility specialist is a doctor (gynecologist) specializing in disorders of fertility.

A neonatal-perinatologist is a doctor specializing in care of the newborn.

A nephrologist is a doctor specializing in the evaluation and treatment of diseases and disorders of the kidney, such as nephritis, kidney failure, and kidney stones. Problems that may lead to referral include blood in the urine, abnormalities on blood tests, urine tests, and scans that indicate a possible kidney problem.

A neurologist is a doctor of the brain and nervous system who diagnoses and treats diseases and disorders such as stroke, multiple sclerosis, nerve damage, neuropathy, movement disorders like Parkinson's, seizures, brain tumors, headaches, dementia, muscular dystrophy, and infections of the brain or spine. Symptoms that may prompt evaluation by a neurologist include muscle weakness, back pain, changes in vision, headaches, numbness or tingling, "spells," tremors, changes in thinking or speech, vertigo, difficulty with balance, personality changes, and nerve pain.

A neuroopthalmologist is an ophthalmologist (eye doctor) who specializes in diseases and disorders of the nervous system of the eye. Symptoms that may prompt referral include double vision, blurred vision, blind spots, nystagmus (rapid eye movements), and migraines.

An oncologist is a doctor trained in internal medicine who specializes in the evaluation and treatment of cancer.

An opthalmologist is a doctor specializing in the evaluation and treatment of diseases of the eye, such as cataracts, glaucoma, iritis, uveitis, conjunctivitis, corneal ulcers, injuries to any part of the eye, retinal tears, and eye tumors. Symptoms that may prompt referral include a change in vision or loss of vision, headache, excessive tearing, and dry eyes.

An otolaryngologist: ENT (see above).

A doctor of physical medicine and rehabilitation is one specializing in the evaluation and treatment of physical debilities caused by injury, illness, or disease.

A psychiatrist is a doctor who diagnoses, treats, and prevents mental illness. A psychiatrist can prescribe medication, whereas a psychologist cannot. Symptoms that may prompt referral include anxiety, changed sleep patterns, nightmares, excessive crying spells, depression, inability to concentrate, prolonged grief, and hallucinations.

A *urologist* is a doctor who diagnoses and treats diseases and disorders of the male genital or urinary tract and female urinary tract, as well as surgical diseases of the adrenal glands. A urologist treats infections of the bladder, kidneys, or urethra (urethritis), venereal disease in men, kidney and bladder stones, cancer of the male genitourinary or female urinary system, kidney failure, prostate problems, and male fertility problems. Symptoms that may prompt evaluation by a urologist include incontinence (inability to hold urine), difficulty with urination or male sexual function, pain above the pubic bone, blood in the urine, and back pain.

A *pulmonologist (doctor of pulmonary disease)* is a doctor specializing in the evaluation and treatment of diseases of the lungs, such as asthma, emphysema, bronchiolitis, occupational lung diseases, bronchitis, pneumonia, sarcoidosis, and lung infections. Symptoms that may prompt referral include cough, wheezing, shortness of breath, coughing up blood, chest pain, X-ray evidence of fluid in or around the lungs or a spot in the lung, and tuberculosis.

A *rheumatologist* is a doctor specializing in diseases of the joints or diseases of inflammation, such as rheumatoid arthritis, systemic lupus erythematosis (lupus, SLE), polymyalgia rheumatica, spondylitis, arthropathy (joint disease) related to cancer, gout, joint infection, and degenerative arthritis. Symptoms that may prompt referral include joint pain, swelling, heat, redness, tenderness, or stiffness and bone or muscle pain.

A *urologist* (see *urologic surgeon* under surgical specialties).

DIAGNOSTIC SPECIALTIES

These specialists are doctors trained in the use of technology for the diagnosis and, sometimes, the treatment of diseases.

A *doctor of nuclear medicine* is one specializing in the use of radionuclides (radioactive substances) for the diagnosis and treatment of diseases such as cancer, thyroid disorders, arthritis, and osteomyelitis (bone infection). Problems that may prompt referral include a nodule in the thyroid, an enlarged thyroid, abnormalities of thyroid blood tests, persistent bone pain, and persistent drainage of a skin wound.

A *pathologist* is a doctor who diagnoses disease by looking at tissue.

A *radiologist* is a doctor who diagnoses disease through interpretation of X rays (including CAT scans, MRI or NMR scans, and angiograms) or sonograms. Some radiologists are trained to do needle biopsies under X-ray guidance or to treat disease by administering medication under X-ray or sonographic guidance.

SURGICAL SPECIALTIES

Surgeons are doctors who are trained in the use of surgery to diagnose or treat disease. Oftentimes their training includes a year or more of general internal medicine or other nonsurgical training. They know when surgery is or is not the best approach to diagnosing or treating a particular problem. A general surgeon is trained to evaluate and treat most common disorders or diseases that require surgical intervention.

A *cardiovascular surgeon* is one who specializes in the repair of the heart or vessels of circulation, such as coronary artery disease (hardening of the arteries that feed the heart), aortic dissection or aneurysm, abdominal aneurysm, peripheral vascular disease (blockage of the vessels to the arms, legs, intestines, or other organ), and abnormal heart valves.

A *colorectal surgeon* is one who specializes in the repair of the colon or rectum following injury, illness, or disease. Many colorectal surgeons perform follow-up colonoscopy when indicated.

A *facial plastic surgeon* is one who specializes in reconstruction and repair of facial abnormalities.

A *neurosurgeon* is one who specializes in surgical repair of the nervous system and surrounding structures. Neurosurgeons operate on slipped disks, bone spurs, and brain and spinal tumors.

An *orthopedic surgeon* is a doctor who evaluates and treats diseases and disorders of the locomotor structures of the body (bones, joints, muscles, ligaments, cartilage), such as bone fractures, bone spurs, fasciitis, shin splints, separated shoulders, and dislocated hips.

A *plastic surgeon* is one specializing in the restoration, repair, or reconstruction of a body structure.

A *thoracic surgeon* is one specializing in surgery of the chest.

A *urologic surgeon (urologist)* is one specializing in the diagnosis and treatment of diseases and disorders of the male and female urinary tract and male genital tract, such as prostate infections, kidney infections, kidney stones, and a blocked urinary system. Symptoms that may prompt referral include blood in the urine, back pain, impotence, and difficulty in urinating.

A *vascular surgeon* is one specializing in the repair and reconstruction of blood and lymph vessels.

ONCOLOGY SPECIALISTS

A *gynecologic oncologist* is a doctor specializing in the evaluation and treatment of cancer of the reproductive organs, such as ovaries, fallopian tubes, uterus, and cervix.

A *medical oncologist* is a doctor trained in internal medicine who specializes in the evaluation and treatment of cancer.

A *radiation oncologist* is a doctor specializing in the treatment of cancer with radiation.

A *surgical oncologist* is a surgeon specializing in the surgical approach to problems due to cancer or its treatment.

NONPHYSICIAN PROFESSIONALS

A *charge nurse* is the head nurse.

A *clinical nurse specialist* is a registered nurse with an additional master's degree in nursing. He or she has particular competence in a special area.

A *graduate nurse* is a nurse who has graduated from nursing school but has not yet taken or passed the certification exams.

A *licensed practical nurse (LPN)* is a nurse who has graduated from a school of practical nursing and has passed the board examination.

A *registered nurse (RN)* is a nurse who has graduated from a state-approved school of nursing and is board-certified.

A *special nurse* is a private duty nurse.

A *student nurse* is a person enrolled in a school of nursing.

An *occupational therapist (OT)* is a professional who helps people whose ability to function independently is limited because of physical limitations. Occupational therapists use therapeutic activities and exercises to help people become more independent in activities of daily living.

A *medical assistant (MA)* is a person who assists a physician with administrative or technical duties. A medical assistant can be certified (CMA) by the American Association of Medical Assistants by completing an approved program and passing competency exams.

A *nurse anesthetist* is a registered nurse (RN) who administers anesthesia to patients.

A *nurse practitioner* is a registered nurse (RN) with special training in the care of certain types of patients where the emphasis is on primary care.

A *physician's assistant* is a person who is specially trained to perform tasks usually done by a physician. All work done by a physician's assistant is supervised by a physician.

A *physical therapist (PT)* is a professional who assists in the examination, testing, and treatment of physically disabled persons. Physical therapists' techniques include special exercises, applications of heat or cold, sonar waves, ultraviolet waves, and massages.

A *psychologist* is a professional trained in psychological analysis, therapy, and/or research. He or she can advise regarding the indication for medication but cannot prescribe medications.

A *social worker* is a professional whose goal is to enhance and maintain psychosocial functioning of individuals, families, and small groups. Hospital social workers assess the home situation, finances, and community resources, as well as social and emotional factors specifically related to the patient's medical condition, and then take action to solve any problems. Social workers are trained to provide counseling and psychotherapy. In the hospital setting, they assist with discharge plans.

DOCTORS IN TRAINING

A *medical student* is a college graduate who is in medical school. Medical students are often referred to as "Doctor X, medical student," or "Student Doctor X," but sometimes as "Doctor X." The name tag will not have an "M.D." after the name. You may encounter the services of medical students when you are a patient in a teaching hospital, the outpatient clinic, or your doctor's private office. All work done by a medical student is overseen by a licensed physician. Student doctors cannot prescribe medication or treatment without a physician's approval and cosignature. You have a right to refuse to be evaluated by medical students without compromising your care. Willingness to be evaluated by medical students contributes to the knowledge and experience of these future doctors.

An intern is a medical doctor who has graduated from medical school and is in his or her first year of postgraduate training.

A resident is a medical doctor who has graduated from medical school and is in at least his or her second year of postgraduate training.

A chief resident is a medical doctor who has graduated from medical school, has completed a residency training program, and is doing an extra year as the resident in charge of the other residents.

A fellow is a medical doctor who has graduated from medical school, has completed a residency training program, and is in a specialty training program.

APPENDIX V

Your Personal Medical Records

A folder or three-ring notebook containing all your important medical information provides you and your family with a valuable resource. Specifics get confused or forgotten with time, even basic information such as the name of your oncologist or surgeon, or your treatments. Information that is recorded immediately is accurate and available for retrieval at a moment's notice.

MEDICATION LIST

Set up a medication list now, and update it regularly. Keep handy an extra copy of a written list of your current medications, including all prescription and nonprescription medicines. Indicate anything you are taking for the prevention of recurrent cancer, pain control, sleep, bowel regularity, depression, fatigue, weight loss or gain, or medical conditions unrelated to your cancer (high blood pressure, diabetes, elevated cholesterol, and so on). Take this list with you every time you go for checkups, consultations, or emergency room visits.

If you have ongoing or intermittent problems, a perpetual medication list (a constantly updated list) keeps track of the start and stop dates of all of your medications. This is especially important if different doctors prescribe medications for you.

A written list makes it easier for you and your health care team to make sure that your medications are factored into the evaluation of any problem and optimized for your current condition. It also safeguards against your receiving medication that is ill advised in light of one of your other medications, drug allergies, or medical conditions. This is especially important when you see many different doctors. Finally, it makes it easier and safer for a new doctor to care for you when your regular doctor is not available. In the event of an emergency, your family's access to the list will ensure that this vital information is available and accurate.

A sample medication list follows. Copy it, or devise your own. Be sure to indicate your name, date of birth, and drug allergies on top. Include the names of all of your medications, the dosages taken (amount taken each time you take the medication), and the times of day you take them.

In addition to your current medication list, make a record of the treatments you received for your cancer (chemotherapy, radiation therapy, biological modifiers, immunological agents, surgery).

LIST OF NAMES AND NUMBERS

Keep a list of the names, telephone numbers, and addresses of all the people in your health care team, as well as offices and organizations whose services you have used. Keep a copy of this list in a convenient place near your telephone. Be sure to include the following people who may have been involved in your care: your medical oncologist(s), radiation oncologist(s), surgeon(s), primary care doctor (internist or family practitioner), consulting specialists (cardiologist, gastroenterologist, gynecologist, and so on), pharmacist, dentist, nurse at the clinic or doctors' offices, private duty nurse, visiting nurse (home health nurse), social worker, physical therapist, occupational therapist, speech therapist, and director of rehabilitation program. Include the following services that were involved in your care: pharmacies (include the closest twenty-four-hour pharmacy), supplier of medical equipment, ambulance, and home nursing care.

You may want to include the names and numbers of people to be called in an emergency, as well as information on the location of your living will and other legal papers.

LISTS OF TESTS

Over the years information about the timing and location of various tests can get mixed up or difficult to retrieve. Keep a log of tests, the dates performed, the location where performed, and the doctor who ordered the test. Some people like to include the test results as well.

You may wish to keep a log of checkups and hospitalizations, including dates and locations. This is most valuable when you are followed by a number of different doctors and when the services provided overlap.

MEDICATIONS LIST

Name

Date of Birth

Weight

DRUG ALLERGIES

Drug	Reaction	Year

Drug	Size	Dose	Times Taken	Start	Stop

MEDICATIONS LIST

Name   Viva Welle

Date of Birth   7/4/66

Weight   140 lbs

DRUG ALLERGIES

Drug	Reaction	Year
Antibiotic "A"	Wheezing	1986
	Fainting	
Pain Medicine "B"	Rash	1989

Drug	Size	Dose	Times Taken	Start	Stop
Multivitamin "Z"		1 tablet	every AM	1986	____
Over-the-counter pain medicine "Y"	500 mg	2 tabs	every 6 hrs as needed	1986	____
Fiber supplement "X"	1/2 oz	1 tbsp	1–2 times per day	1986	____
Asthma sprayer "W"		2 puffs	every 8 hrs	1986	____
Hormone "V"	1 mg	1 tablet	every AM Day 1–25	1990	____
Hormone "U"	10 mg	1/2 tab	every AM Day 16–25	1990	____
Antibiotic "T"	250 mg	1 capsule	every 12 hrs	8/9/93	8/19/93
Cough syrup "S"	15 mg	1–2 tsp	every 4 hrs as needed	8/9/93	8/19/93
Antinausea "R"	25 mg	1/2–1 tablet	every 8 hrs as needed	10/3/93	10/8/93
Sleep medicine "Q"	15 mg	1/2 tablet	before bed as needed	10/10/93	____
Antibiotic "P"	500 mg	1 tablet	every 8 hrs with meals	4/1/94	4/15/94
Antibiotic "P"	250 mg	1 tablet	every 8 hrs with meals	4/16/94	4/23/94

APPENDIX VI

Cancer's Warning Signs

If you show a warning sign for cancer, it does *not* mean that you probably have cancer. A warning sign is a signal that you need to be evaluated for cancer and the many other conditions that cause these symptoms. Have any warning signs checked out as soon as possible in order to

- save you unnecessary worry if the warning sign is due to something that does not need treatment
- get you started on treatment if it is a noncancerous condition that needs attention
- maximize your chances of doing well if you do have cancer

See your doctor as soon as possible if you develop

- a lump or thickening in the breast or elsewhere
- itching, bleeding, or change in the size, shape, or color of a mole or wart
- difficulty in swallowing
- indigestion
- change in bowel or bladder habits
- unusual bleeding or discharge
- a sore that does not heal
- hoarseness or cough
- unexplained weight loss
- unexplained fevers, sweats
- any unexplained change from what is usual for you, especially if the change persists for more than a few days

APPENDIX VII

Specific Steps for Cancer Prevention

- avoid exposure to known cancer-causing substances whenever possible (e.g., tobacco, asbestos)
- eat a varied diet
- eat in moderation
- maintain a desirable weight; avoid obesity
- include fiber in your diet
- eat four to six helpings of fruits and vegetables daily
- eat cruciferous vegetables (cabbage family)
- eat a low-fat diet (limit fat to 30 percent of your total intake)
- have carbohydrates constitute 55 percent of your caloric intake
- consume foods rich in complex carbohydrates
- minimize salt-cured, smoked, and nitrite-cured foods
- avoid excessive consumption of alcohol
- avoid too much refined sugar
- avoid excessive exposure to the sun
- use a sunscreen with SPF of at least 15
- stay well nourished and physically fit
- if you have a baby, nurse the baby
- delay the onset of sexual activity
- maintain a monogamous relationship
- use barrier contraception
- have precancerous lesions removed (precancerous moles, adenomatous colon polyps) or monitored closely (leukoplakia of the mouth)
- avoid high-dose estrogen; avoid unopposed estrogen
- treat undescended testicles

APPENDIX VIII

Specific Cancer Screening

Breast	• BSE (Breast self-exam) • physician exam • mammography
Cervical	• physical exam • PAP smears
Colorectal (bowel)	• digital rectal exam • fecal occult blood testing (FOB) • proctosigmoidoscopy ("scope test")
Endometrial (uterine)	• physical exam • baseline endometrial aspiration at menopause
Head and Neck	• physical exam
Lung	• no general screening for nonsmokers • chest X ray for heavy smokers
Melanoma	• skin self-exam • physican skin exam
Prostate	• digital rectal exam • PSA (blood test)
Testicular	• testicular self-exam • physician testicular exam

Index

—